DRUGS FOR BUGS

2003

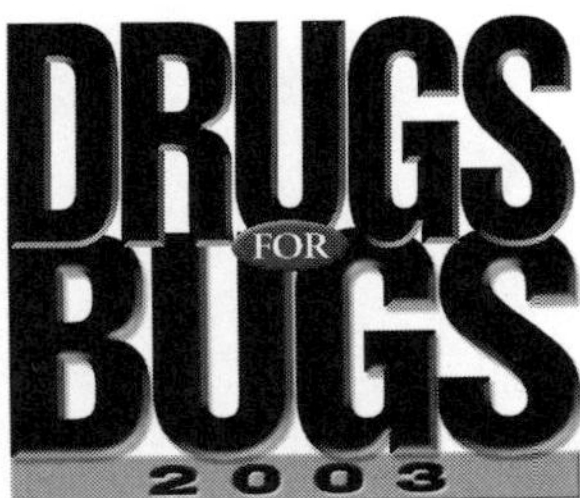

The Saint-Frances Guide to Outpatient Antimicrobial Therapy

Paul D. Baker, ARNP, MSN, BSN, BS
Antibiotic Research Clinic, VA Puget Sound Health Care System
Family Nurse Practitioner, South Kitsap Family Care Clinic
Port Orchard, Washington

Christopher T. Hoey, PharmD, BCPS
Clinical Pharmacist, Head, Program for Intravenous Outpatient Therapy
VA Puget Sound Health Care System, Clinical Instructor, University of Washington, School of Pharmacy, Seattle, Washington

Benjamin A. Lipsky, MD, FACP, FIDSA
Professor of Medicine, University of Washington, School of Medicine
Director, General Internal Medicine Clinic, Director, Antibiotic Research Clinic
VA Puget Sound Health Care System

Series Editor: Sanjay Saint, MD, MPH
Associate Professor of Medicine
Research Scientist, Ann Arbor VA Medical Center
Director, Patient Safety Enhancement Program
University of Michigan Health System, Ann Arbor, Michigan

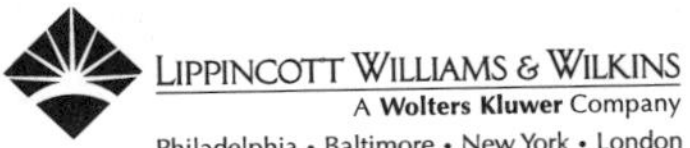

Editor: Neil Marquardt
Managing Editor: Daniel Pepper
Marketing Manager: Scott Lavine
Project Editor: Paula C. Williams
Designer: Doug Smock
Compositor: Techbooks
Printer: Malloy, Inc.

351 West Camden Street
Baltimore, Maryland 21201-2436 USA

530 Walnut Street
Philadelphia, Pennsylvania 19106-3621 USA

The publisher is not responsible (as a matter of product liability, negligence, or otherwise) for any injury resulting from any material contained herein. This publication contains information relating to general principles of medical care which should not be construed as specific instructions for individual patients. Manufacturers' product information and package inserts should be reviewed for current information, including contraindications, dosages, and precautions.

Printed in the United States of America

Library of Congress Cataloging-in-Publication Data

LOC data is available: 0-7817-4197-1

The publishers have made every effort to trace the copyright holders for borrowed material. If they have inadvertently overlooked any, they will be pleased to make the necessary arrangements at the first opportunity.

To purchase additional copies of this book call our customer service department at **(800) 638-3030** or fax orders to (301) 824-7390. International customers should call **(301) 714-2324.**

Visit Lippincott Williams & Wilkins on the Internet: http://www.lww.com. Lippincott Williams & Wilkins customer service representatives are available from 8:30 am to 6:00 pm, EST, Monday through Friday, for telephone access.

02 03 04

1 2 3 4 5 6 7 8 9 10

To Ben and Sanjay: two friends and mentors who always gave me support and guidance. To David, gone but not forgotten. To my wife Lyn, who gave me the most precious gift of all, Ethan.

Paul D. Baker

To Nolan, Gareth, and Patty with gratitude for sharing my enthusiasm for this project.

Christopher T. Hoey

To Donna, with thanks for your constant support and encouragement.

Benjamin A. Lipsky

Table of Contents

List of Drugs

Preface

This guide is designed to provide the clinician with a quick and convenient reference for antimicrobial therapy in the outpatient setting. The information contained in *Drugs for Bugs: The Saint-Frances Guide to Outpatient Antimicrobial Therapy* was compiled from many sources, including published literature, drug package inserts, professional guidelines and consultation with local infectious disease and pharmacotherapy experts. We have spared no effort in ensuring that this information is up-to-date and accurate. Although we have chosen not to list references (to save space), the reader can be assured that all recommendations are as evidence-based as possible. The accuracy of this guide cannot, however, be guaranteed and it should complement but not substitute for clinical experience, expert consultation, data provided by the drug manufacturers and constant perusal of new medical literature. Note that some drug doses or indications may not be FDA approved at this time, but we believe they are appropriate and represent current practice standards.

How to use this guide – There are other handbooks of antimicrobial therapy, but we have tried to make this one the most practical, quickest and easiest to use. While most of the infections covered are bacterial, we also describe therapy for the most common fungal, viral and parasitic diseases seen in outpatients.

Infectious diseases or syndromes are arranged anatomically, from the head downwards. Thus, otitis media is near the front of the guide, pneumonia about the middle and urinary tract infections toward the end. Within body site categories, sub-categories of infections are arranged alphabetically. We provide recommended doses, modified when necessary for age, body weight, etc. Relevant information on drug formulations, how and when to take the drugs (especially in regard to food), important adverse effects and precautions, and drug prices are provided for each agent. Thus, everything the clinician and patient need to know to optimize antimicrobial therapy is provided in one easily accessible place.

Cost of therapy - The drug prices indicated in this guide are derived from Average Wholesale Prices (AWP) quoted in the Redbook© 2001. Actual prices paid by the consumer may differ from the price indicated; in many cases, they may be lower. The prices quoted are intended to provide a comparison among otherwise similar options and a general estimate of the potential cost to the consumer. In many cases, the cost of a brand name product will greatly exceed that of a generic.

Key:

<$ = <$10.00
$ = <$20.00
$$ = <$40.00
$$$ = <$60.00
$$$$ = ≤$80.00
>$$$$ = >$80.00

Choice of therapy - For each infection listed, the recommended therapy was based on several factors, including proven clinical efficacy, drug safety, cost of therapy, professional guidelines, literature reviews and well-established protocols. All possible medication choices are not listed for each infection; rather we have chosen to recommend only those therapies that are most widely accepted. When there is a clear drug of choice (DOC) that medication is underlined. Otherwise, the various potentially appropriate medications are listed, in most cases, alphabetically. The most frequent or clinically important pathogens are listed on parenthesis for many of the infectious syndromes.

Oral contraceptives and antibiotics - Current evidence indicates that rifampin and griseofulvin may induce hepatic enzymes, resulting in enhanced elimination of ethinyl estradiol and reduced effectiveness of oral contraceptives. Studies with other antibiotics, in small groups of women, have not shown that they significantly impair the activity of oral contraceptives. However, there appears to be large interindividual variation in the effect of certain antibiotics on ethinyl estradiol levels. Administration of some antibiotics, notably penicillins and tetracyclines, may result in significantly decreased plasma levels of ethinyl estradiol in a few women. Since it is not possible to identify which women may be at risk of contraceptive failure we advise caution in using of antibiotics in women taking oral contraceptives. Additional methods of barrier contraception during, and for up to a week after completion of antibiotic therapy, may be prudent.

References:

1. Dickinson, BD, Altman RD, Nielsen NH, Sterling ML, From the Council on Scientific Affairs, American Medical Association. Drug interactions between oral contraceptives and antibiotics. Obset Gynecol 2001 Nov;98(5 Pt 1):853-60.
2. Weaver K, Glasier A. Interaction between broad-spectrum antibiotics and the combination oral contraceptive pill. A literature review. Contraception 1999 Feb;59(2):71-8.
3. Weisberg E. Interactions between oral contraceptives and antifungals/antibacterials. Is contraceptive failure the result? Clin Pharmacokinet 1999 May;36(5):309-13.

Beta lactam drug allergy - Patients who have demonstrated an allergic reaction to a penicillin antibiotic have a low risk (approximately 7-11%) of also being allergic to cephalosporin antibiotics. They may, however, have an eight-fold greater risk of being allergic to cephalosporins than patients who have not shown a previous reaction to penicillins. Previous allergic reaction to a penicillin or cephalosporin is the most important risk factor for predicting a future reaction to drugs from these classes. In this guide, those drugs which are generally considered to be safe to administer to patients with a previous allergic reaction to a penicillin or cephalosporin are indicated with a (*).

Reference: Kelkar PS, Li T-C. Cephalosporin allergy. N Engl J Med 2001;345(11):804-809.

Common respiratory infections – Over half of all antibiotic courses in the United States are for sinusitis, pharyngitis, and bronchitis. Because a substantial proportion (probably the majority) of these infections are not caused by bacteria, and the efficacy of antibiotic therapy for many of these infections is not well documented, there is considerable controversy about appropriate treatment. We support avoiding antibiotic therapy when it is not necessary, but have provided guidance on appropriate choices when it is.

Renal clearance - Drugs which are eliminated significantly by the kidney may require dose modifications in patients with impaired renal function. The authors provide general guidelines in the therapeutic section and more specific suggestions in the "List of Drugs" section. An estimate of creatinine clearance (CrCl) can be obtained using the formula:

CrCl (males) = (140 − patient age in years) × (weight in Kg)/Serum Creatinine × 72

CrCl (females) = above value × 0.85

FDA Pregnancy Safety Categories:

A = Safety has been established. Minimal or no risk.

B = Animal studies show no risk; human studies are inadequate.

C = Animal studies show a risk; human studies are inadequate.

D = Evidence of human risk exists.

X = High risk to fetus.

? = Safety is unknown

Lac: Is this drug safe to use during lactation (breast feeding)

* = Can be used for penicillin allergic patients.

Abbreviations

Q12H - two times daily
Caps - capsules
CrCl - Creatinine Clearance
  CrCl (males) = (140-patient age in years) × (weight in Kg)/Serum Creatinine × 72
  CrCl (females) = above value × 0.85
g - gram
GI - gastrointestinal
gm - gram
IA - intraarticular
IV - intravenous
kg - kilogram (approximately 2.2 pounds)
lb - pound (approximately 0.45 kilograms)
LFT - liver function tests
max - maximum
mL - milliliter
NTE - no to exceed
OTC - over the counter or available without a prescription
PO - by mouth or orally
PRN - as needed or if needed
Q6H - four times daily
Q12H - every twelve hours
Q6H - every six hours
Q8H - every eight hours
Q24H - once daily
qHS - every night at bedtime
RUQ - right upper quadrant
SC - subcutaneous
SrCr - serum creatinine
SQ - subcutaneous
Susp - suspension
Tabs - tablets
tbsp - tablespoonful (approximately 15 mL or one-half ounce)
Q8H - three times daily
tsp - teaspoonful (approximately 5 mL)
WBC - white blood cell

DRUGS FOR BUGS

2003

Drug, Its Forms and Dosage Increments	Children and Adult Dosages and Instructions	Information and Important Side Effects
HEAD – Lice (*Pediculus humanus capitis*)		
<u>Permethrin</u> **(OTC)** (Nix Cream Rinse® 1%) Pregnancy: B; Lactation: Unk **Cream Rinse 1%** 60-mL bottle - <$ **Cream 5% (Rx Only):** For scabies only.	**Children >2 months:** **Rinse:** Wash hair, towel dry, saturate hair with Nix, and rinse after 10 minutes. Remove remaining nits with nit comb. One treatment eliminates infestations. Repeat only if live lice are seen after 7 days. Wash bedding and all clothing in hot water. Vacuum furniture and dispose of bag.	**Important side effects:** Mild temporary itching or erythema. Avoid contact with mucous membranes. Contraindicated if allergic to chrysanthemum flower.
Pyrethrins/piperonyl butoxide (OTC) (RID®, A-200®, Pronto®) Other products available Pregnancy: C; Lactation: Unk **Bottles:** 60 mL, 120 mL, 240 mL 120 mL (two applications) - <$	**Children and Adult:** Apply to dry hair. After 10 minutes, wash hair, rinse thoroughly. Comb out hair with nit comb. Repeat in 7-10 days. Wash bedding and all clothing in hot water. Vacuum furniture and dispose of bag.	**Important side effects:** Burning, pruritus. Contraindicated if allergic to ragweed or chrysanthemum flower.
HEAD – Tinea Capitis, Fungal (*Trichophyton tonsurans, Microsporum canis*)		
<u>Griseofulvin microsize</u> (Grifulvin-V®, Fulvicin-U/F®) Pregnancy: C; Lactation: Unk Generics available **Tabs:** 250 mg, 500 mg **Caps:** 250 mg **Oral Susp:** 125 mg/5 mL 120 mL - $31.10	**Children:** 10-20 mg/kg/day in one or two divided doses (max 500 mg/day). **Using 125 mg/5 mL @ 10 mg/kg/day** 5 kg (11 lb) = 2 mL Q24H 7.5 kg (16 lb) = 3 mL Q24H 10 kg (22 lb) = 4 mL Q24H 12.5 kg (28 lb) = 5 mL (1tsp) Q24H 15 kg (33 lb) = 6 mL Q24H	**Food:** With food, especially fatty meal, to increase absorption. **Important side effects:** Rash, urticaria, headache, dizziness, hepatotoxicity (rare). Avoid prolonged exposure to sunlight and avoid alcohol.

Adult 4-6 weeks - $$–$$$	20 kg (44 lb) = 8 mL Q24H 25 kg (55 lb) = 10 mL (2 tsp) Q24H or 250-mg tab/cap Q24H Treat until hair regrows (usually 4-8 weeks). **Adult:** 500 mg once daily or 250 mg twice daily for 4-6 weeks.	
Itraconazole* (Sporanox®) Pregnancy: C; Lactation: Unsafe **Caps:** 100 mg - >$$$$ **Oral Solution:** 100 mg/10 mL (150 mL)	**Children:** 5 mg/kg/day (max 100 mg/day) once daily for 4-6 weeks. Limited information on use in children. **Using 100 mg/10 mL @ 5 mg/kg/day** 5 kg (11 lb) = 2.5 mL Q24H 10 kg (22 lb) = 5 mL (1 tsp) Q24H 15 kg (33 lb) = 7.5 mL Q24H 25 kg (55 lb) = 10 mL (2 tsp) Q24H or 100-mg cap **Adult:** 100 mg daily for 4-6 weeks.	**Food:** Avoid grapefruit products. Take capsules with food. Take oral solution on an empty stomach. Not well absorbed with acid-suppressing drugs. **Important side effects:** Advise patient to report any signs of liver failure: anorexia, nausea, vomiting, RUQ discomfort, jaundice, ascites. **Caution:** May cause hepatitis. Use with caution in persons with history of liver disease. Consider periodic liver function tests. May cause or contribute to congestive heart failure or cardiac dysrhythmias. Use with caution in persons with history of cardiac disease. Use is contraindicated in any patient taking cisapride, dofetilide, quinidine, midazolam, triazolam, pimozide, lovastatin, or simvastatin. Not *(continued)*

Drug, Its Forms and Dosage Increments	Children and Adult Dosages and Instructions	Information and Important Side Effects
		well absorbed with acid-suppressing drug. Has caused bone defects and changes in tooth appearance in rats; implications for humans are not established.
Terbinafine* (Lamisil®) Pregnancy: B; Lactation: Unsafe **Tabs:** 250 mg - Adult - >$$$$	**Children:** Difficult to give to children <20 kg. **<20 kg:** 62.5 mg once daily for 4-8 weeks. **20-40 kg:** 125 mg once daily for 4-8 weeks. **≥40 kg and Adult:** 250 mg PO daily for 4-8 weeks. Baseline LFT should be obtained.	**Food:** With or without meals. **Important side effects:** Advise patient to report any signs of liver failure: anorexia, nausea, vomiting, RUQ discomfort, jaundice, ascites.
Fluconazole* (Diflucan®) Pregnancy: C; Lactation: Unsafe **Tabs:** 50 mg, 100 mg, 150 mg, 200 mg **Oral Susp:** 10 mg/mL, 40 mg/mL	**Children:** 8 mg/kg (NTE 200 mg/day) once per week for 8-12 weeks. **40 mg/mL @ 8 mg/kg** 10 kg (22 lb) = 2 mL (80 mg) 15 kg (33 lb) = 3 mL (120 mg) 20 kg (44 lb) = 4 mL (160 mg) 40 kg (88 lb) = Use adult dose. **Adult:** 200-300 mg once per week for 8-12 weeks.	**Food:** With or without meals. **Important side effects:** Advise patient to report any signs of liver failure: anorexia, nausea, vomiting, RUQ discomfort, jaundice, ascites.
Selenium sulfide* (Selsun®, Exsel®) Generics available	**Children and Adult:** Shampoo twice weekly until resolved (average 2 weeks). Leave in hair for 2-3 minutes, then rinse and repeat.	**Important side effects:** May irritate skin and discolor hair or jewelry. Rinse thoroughly after use.

Pregnancy: C; Lactation: Unk
Shampoo 1% (OTC)
Selsun Blue®
Shampoo and Lotion 2.5%:
Rx and OTC - 240-mL bottle - <$

Wash hands after use. Avoid contact with eye(s) and inflamed skin.
May be useful adjunct to griseofulvin; unlikely to be effective alone.

EYE(S) – Conjunctivitis, Acute Bacterial (*Staphylococcus aureus, Streptococcus pneumoniae, Haemophilus influenzae*)

Erythromycin*
(Ilotycin®)
Generics available
Pregnancy: B; Lactation: Safe
Ophth Oint 0.5%: 3.5 g - <$

Children and Adult: Apply ribbon to lower lid of affected eye(s) every 3-4 hours while awake. Continue for 7-10 days.

Important side effects: Blurring of vision.

Polymyxin B + Trimethoprim*
(Polytrim®)
Pregnancy: C; Lactation: Unk
Ophth Sol: 10,000 U polymyxin/1 mg/mL trimethoprim
10-mL bottle - $

Children >2 months to Adult: Apply 1-2 drops to affected eye(s) every 3 hours while awake. Continue for 7-10 days. Max 6 gtt/day.

Polymyxin B + Bacitracin*
(Polysporin®)
Generics available
Pregnancy: C; Lactation: Unk
Ophth Oint: 3.5-g tube - $

Children >2 months to Adult: Apply ribbon to lower lid of affected eye(s) every 3-4 hours while awake for acute infection, or two to three times daily for moderate infection for 7-10 days.

Important side effects: Blurring of vision.

Sulfacetamide
(Sodium Sulamyd®, Bleph-10®, Sulf-10®)
Generics available

Children and Adult: Instill 1-2 drops to lower conjunctival sac of affected eye(s) every 1-3 hours while awake for 7-10 days.

Important side effects: Burning and sensitivity to light. Ointment may cause blurring of vision.

(continued)

Drug, Its Forms and Dosage Increments	Children and Adult Dosages and Instructions	Information and Important Side Effects
Pregnancy: C; Lactation: Unsafe **Soln:** 10%, 15%, 30% **Oint:** 10%	OR ½-inch ribbon on lower conjunctival sac of affected eye(s) 4 times daily and at bedtime for 7-10 days.	
A Fluoroquinolone Ciloxan® (Ciprofloxacin) Quixin® (Levofloxacin) Ocuflox® (Ofloxacin) Pregnancy: C; Lactation: Unsafe **Ophth Sol:** 2.5 mL, 5 mL, 10 mL - $$$	**Adult:** Instill 1-2 drops into affected eye(s) every 2 hours while awake for two days, then every 4 hours while awake for 5 days.	

EYE(S) - Conjunctivitis, Chlamydial - Newborns (*Chlamydia trachomatis*)

Drug, Its Forms and Dosage Increments	Children and Adult Dosages and Instructions	Information and Important Side Effects
Erythromycin Estolate Suspension* (Ilosone®) Generics available **Oral Susp:** 125 mg/5 mL, 250 mg/5 mL	**Neonate:** 50 mg/kg/day in divided doses four times daily for 10-14 days. **125 mg/5 mL @ 50 mg/kg/day** 4-5 kg (9-11 lb) = 2 mL Q6H 5.5-7 kg (12-15 lb) = 3 mL Q6H 7-8 kg (16-18 lb) = 4 mL Q6H	**Food:** With or without meals. Take with food if causes GI upset. **Important side effects:** GI upset, hepatitis.

EYE(S) - Conjunctivitis, Chlamydial - Adult (*Chlamydia trachomatis*)

Comment: Consider referring sex partner for evaluation and treatment.

Drug, Its Forms and Dosage Increments	Children and Adult Dosages and Instructions	Information and Important Side Effects
Doxycycline* (Vibramycin®) Generics available	**Children ≥8 years and Adult:** 100 mg twice daily for 7 days.	**Food:** May take with food if GI upset occurs. Take 1 hour before or 2 hours after antacids, iron, milk, or other dairy

Pregnancy: D; Lactation: Unsafe **Tabs:** 50 mg, 100 mg - <$ **Caps:** 50 mg, 100 mg - <$		products. Take with full glass of water to prevent esophagitis. **Important side effects:** Photosensitivity, esophagitis. May discolor fingernails.
Azithromycin* (Zithromax®) Pregnancy: B; Lactation: Unk **Tabs:** 250 mg - $$ **Powder for Oral Suspension:** 1-g packet - $$	**Children ≥45 kg and Adult:** 1 g PO × 1 dose.	**Food:** 1-g powder packet for oral suspension and tablets without regard to food. **Important side effects:** Nausea, diarrhea, elevated LFTs.
Erythromycin Base* (E-Mycin®, Eryc®) Pregnancy: B; Lactation: Safe **Tabs:** 250 mg, 333 mg, 500 mg - <$ **Caps:** 250 mg	**Children ≥40 kg (88 lb) and Adult:** 500 mg four times daily for 7 days. Less effective than doxycycline or azithromycin. Consider retesting 3 weeks after therapy.	**Food:** May take with or without meals. Take with food if causes GI upset. **Important side effects:** GI upset, hepatitis. Drug interactions may be significant.

EYE(S) – Conjunctivitis, Chlamydial – Pregnant Woman (*Chlamydia trachomatis*)

Azithromycin* (Zithromax®) Pregnancy: B; Lactation: Unk **Tabs:** 250 mg - $$ **Powder for Oral Suspension:** 1 g - $$	**Adolescent and Adult:** 1 g PO × 1.	**Food:** 1-g powder packet for oral suspension and tablets without regard to food. **Important side effects:** Nausea, diarrhea, elevated LFTs.
Erythromycin Base* (E-Mycin®, Eryc®) Generics available	**Adolescent and Adult:** 500 mg four times daily for 7 days **OR** 250 mg four times daily for 14 days if GI upset.	**Food:** May take with or without meals. Take with food if causes GI upset.

(continued)

EYE(S) – Conjunctivitis, Chlamydial – Pregnant Woman (*Chlamydia trachomatis*)

Drug, Its Forms and Dosage Increments	Children and Adult Dosages and Instructions	Information and Important Side Effects
Pregnancy: B; Lactation: Safe **Tabs:** 250 mg, 333 mg, 500 mg **Caps:** 250 mg	This drug is less effective than azithromycin. Consider retesting 3 weeks after therapy.	**Important side effects:** GI upset, hepatitis. Drug interactions may be significant.

EYE(S) – Conjunctivitis, Gonococcal – Children <45 kg (*Neisseria gonorrhoeae*)

Drug, Its Forms and Dosage Increments	Children and Adult Dosages and Instructions	Information and Important Side Effects
Ceftriaxone (Rocephin®) Pregnancy: B; Lactation: Unk **Vials:** 250 mg, 500 mg, 1,000 mg 1 g - $$$	**Children <45 kg:** 25-50 mg/kg (max 125 mg) IM × 1 dose. Treat mother and her partner(s).	**Important side effects:** Pain at injection site.

EYE(S) – Conjunctivitis, Gonococcal – Children ≥45 kg and Adults (*Neisseria gonorrhoeae*)

Drug, Its Forms and Dosage Increments	Children and Adult Dosages and Instructions	Information and Important Side Effects
Ceftriaxone (Rocephin®) Pregnancy: B; Lactation: Unk **Vials:** 250 mg, 500 mg, 1,000 mg 1 g - $$$	**Children ≥45 kg and Adults:** 1 g IM × 1 dose. Lavage affected eye(s) with saline once.	**Important side effects:** Pain at injection site.

EYE(S) – Hordeolum – Stye (*Staphylococcus aureus*)

Comment: No antibiotic treatment needed unless serious, e.g., if cellulitis or conjunctivitis is present. Warm soaks are usually sufficient.

EYE(S) – Orbital Cellulitis (*Streptococcus pneumoniae, Staphylococcus aureus*, Group A *Streptococcus, Haemophilus influenzae*)

Comment: Consult ophthalmologist ASAP. Will likely require parenteral antibiotic therapy.

EARS – Otitis Externa, Acute – "Swimmer's ear" (*Pseudomonas aeruginosa, Staphylococcus aureus*)

Drug	Dosage	Comments
Acetic acid 2%* (VoSol HC® otic) Generics available Pregnancy: Unk; Lactation: Unk **Sol:** 15-mL bottle - <$	**Children and Adult:** Saturate cotton wick and insert in ear. Apply 3-5 drops to wick every 4-6 hours for 24 hours. Remove wick, then instill 3-5 drops in affected ear(s) three to four times daily for as long as needed.	
Acetic acid 2% + Hydrocortisone 1%* (VoSol HC® otic) Pregnancy: Unk; Lactation: Unk **Sol:** 10-mL bottle - <$	**Children and Adult:** Saturate cotton wick and insert in ear. Apply 3-5 drops to wick every 4-6 hours × 24 hours. Remove wick, then instill 3-5 drops in affected ear(s) three to four times daily for as long as needed.	
Cortisporin® Otic* (Hydrocortisone 1% + polymyxin + neomycin) Generics available Pregnancy: C; Lactation: Unk **Otic Sol and Susp 1%:** 7.5 mL, 10 mL 10-mL bottle - $$	**Children and Adult:** Instill 3-4 drops in affected ear(s) three or four times daily for 5-10 days. Use suspension only for perforated TM.	**Important side effects:** Neomycin is sensitizing in some patients.
Ofloxacin 0.3% Otic Solution (Floxin Otic®) Pregnancy: C; Lactation: Unsafe	**Children 1-12 years:** Instill 5 drops in affected ear(s) twice daily for 10 days. **Children ≥12 years and Adults:** Instill 10 drops in affected ear(s) twice daily for 10 days.	**Important side effects:** May cause ear irritation in some individuals.

(continued)

Drug, Its Forms and Dosage Increments	Children and Adult Dosages and Instructions	Information and Important Side Effects
EARS – Otitis Externa with Cellulitis (*Staphylococcus aureus*)		
Dicloxacillin (Dynapen®) Generics available Pregnancy: B; Lactation: Unk **Caps:** 125 mg, 250 mg, 500 mg **Oral Susp:** 62.5 mg/5 mL 200 mL - $ Adult 10-14 days - $	**Children ≤40 kg:** 25-50 mg/kg/day (NTE 2 g/day) in divided doses every 6 hours for 10-14 days. **62.5 mg/5 mL @ 25 mg/kg/day** (double for 50 mg) 10 kg (22 lb) = 1 tsp (5 mL) Q6H 15 kg (33 lb) = 1½ tsp (7.5 mL) Q6H 20 kg (44 lb) = 2 tsp (10 mL) Q6H 30 kg (66 lb) = 3 tsp (15 mL) Q6H **Children ≥40 kg:** 125-500 mg every 6 hours for 10-14 days. **Adult:** 250-500 mg every 6 hours for 10-14 days.	**Food:** Take 1 hour before or 2 hours after meals. **Important side effects:** Bad taste, GI upset.
Cephalexin (Keflex®) Generics available Pregnancy: B; Lactation: Unk **Tabs:** 250 mg, 500 mg, 1 g **Caps:** 250 mg, 500 mg **Oral Susp:** 125 mg/5 mL, 250 mg/5 mL 250 mg/5 mL Q6H × 10 days - <$ 500 mg PO Q6H × 10 days - $	**Children:** 25-50 mg/kg/day NTE 4 g/day in divided doses four times daily for 10 days. **125 mg/5 mL @ 25 mg/kg/day** (double for 50 mg/kg) 10 kg (22 lb) = ½ tsp (2.5 mL) Q6H 15 kg (33 lb) = ¾ tsp Q6H 20 kg (44 lb) = 1 tsp (5 mL) Q6H **250 mg/5 mL @ 25 mg/kg/day** (double for 50 mg/kg) 20 kg (44 lb) = ½ tsp (2.5 mL) Q6H	**Food:** May take with food if GI upset occurs. **Important side effects:** GI upset, diarrhea. **Reduce dose in renal disease (CrCl <40 mL/min).**

40 kg (88 lb) = 1 tsp (5 mL) Q6H
>40 kg = Use adult dose.
Adult: 250-500 mg PO four times daily for 10 days.

Amoxicillin-clavulanate
(Augmentin®)
Pregnancy: B; Lactation: Unk
Q12H Formulations:
Tabs: 500 mg/125 mg, 875 mg/125 mg
Chewable Tabs:
200 mg/28.5 mg, 400 mg/57 mg
Oral Susp:
200 mg/28.5 mg/5 mL,
400 mg/57 mg/5 mL
Q8H Formulations:
Tabs: 250 mg/125 mg, 500 mg/125 mg
Chewable Tabs:
125 mg/31.25 mg, 250 mg/62.5 mg
Oral Susp:
125 mg/31.25 mg/5 mL,
250 mg/62.5 mg/5 mL
Cost of 10-day course:
Child - $$$ Adult - >$$$$

Neonates and infants ≤3 months:
Use 125 mg/31.25 mg/5 mL suspension. 30 mg/kg/day in divided doses every 12 hours.
Children ≥3 months up to 40 kg:
20-45 mg amoxicillin component/kg/day (max 1600 mg/day) in divided doses two or three times daily for 10-14 days.
Q12H using 200 mg/5 mL susp @ 45 mg/kg/day
9 kg (20 lb) = 1 tsp (5 mL) Q12H
13 kg (29 lb) = 1½ tsp (7.5 mL) Q12H
18 kg (40 lb) = 2 tsp (10 mL) Q12H
Q12H using 400 mg/5 mL susp @ 45 mg/kg/day
18 kg (40 lb) = 1 tsp (5 mL) Q12H
27 kg (59 lb) = 1½ tsp (7.5 mL) Q12H
35 kg (77 lb) = 2 tsp (10 mL) Q12H
>40 kg (88 lb) = Use adult dose (max 875 mg Q12H).
Adult: 500-875 mg PO every 12 hours for 10-14 days.
Note: Q12H dosing may improve compliance compared to Q8H dosing.

Food: Take with food to reduce diarrhea.
Important side effects: Diarrhea (common), nausea, rash. May cause nonallergic maculopapular rash.
Reduce dose in renal disease (CrCl <30 mL/min).

(continued)

Drug, Its Forms and Dosage Increments	Children and Adult Dosages and Instructions	Information and Important Side Effects
	Use amoxicillin component to calculate dosing.	
Clindamycin* (Cleocin®) Generics available Pregnancy: B; Lactation: Unk **Cleocin Caps:** 75 mg, 150 mg, 300 mg **Peds Oral Susp:** 75 mg/5 mL 150 mg/10 mL Q8H × 10 days - $$$ 300 mg PO Q6H × 10 days - $$	**Children: Mild to moderate infections:** 10-15 mg/kg/day (NTE 1.8 g/day) in divided doses 3 times daily for 10-14 days. **Serious infection:** 15-25 mg/kg/day (NTE 1.8 g/day) in divided doses 3 or 4 times daily for 10-14 days. **75 mg/5 mL @ 10 mg/kg/day** (double for 20 mg/kg) 10 kg (22 lb) = 2 mL Q8H 20 kg (44 lb) = 4 mL Q8H 30 kg (66 lb) = 6 mL Q8H 40 kg (88 lb) = 8 mL Q8H >40 kg = Use adult dose. **Adult: Mild to moderate infection:** 150-300 mg PO three or four times daily for 10-14 days. **Serious infection:** 450 mg PO three or four times daily for 10-14 days.	**Food:** With or without meals. Take with full glass of water to prevent esophagitis. **Important side effects:** Diarrhea may be severe. Esophagitis. **May cause severe colitis.** Encourage patient to report severe, persistent, or bloody diarrhea.

EARS – Otitis Externa, Chronic (*Staphylococcus aureus*)

Hydrocortisone 0.5% + Polymyxin B Otic* (Otobiotic®)	**Children and Adult:** Instill 4 drops in affected ear(s) three to four times daily.	

Pregnancy: Unk; Lactation: Unk
Otic Solution: 15 mL

EARS – Otitis Externa, Furuncle (*Staphylococcus aureus*)

Drug	Dosing	Comments
Cephalexin (Keflex®) Generics available Pregnancy: B; Lactation: Unk **Tabs:** 250 mg, 500 mg, 1 g **Caps:** 250 mg, 500 mg **Oral Susp:** 125 mg/5 mL, 250 mg/5 mL 250 mg/5 mL Q6H × 10 days - <$ 500 mg PO Q6H × 10 days - $	**Children**: 25-50 mg/kg/day (max 4 g/day) in divided doses three to four times daily for 10 days. **125 mg/5 mL @ 25 mg/kg/day** (double for 50 mg/kg) 10 kg (22 lb) = ½ tsp (2.5 mL) Q6H 15 kg (33 lb) = ¾ tsp Q6H 20 kg (44 lb) = 1 tsp (5 mL) Q6H **250 mg/5 mL @ 25 mg/kg/day** (double for 50 mg/kg) 20 kg (44 lb) = ½ tsp (2.5 mL) Q6H 40 kg (88 lb) = 1 tsp (5 mL) Q6H >40 kg = Use adult dose. **Adult:** 250-500 mg PO four times daily for 10 days.	**Food:** May take with food if GI upset occurs. **Important side effects:** GI upset, diarrhea. **Reduce dose in renal disease (CrCl <40 mL/min).**
Dicloxacillin (Dynapen®) Generics available Pregnancy: B; Lactation: Unk **Caps:** 125 mg, 250 mg, 500 mg **Oral Susp:** 62.5 mg/5 mL 200 mL - $ Adult 10-14 days - $	**Children ≤40 kg:** 25-50 mg/kg/day (NTE 2 g/day) in divided doses every 6 hours for 10-14 days. **62.5 mg/5 mL @ 25 mg/kg/day** (double for 50 mg) 10 kg (22 lb) = 1 tsp (5 mL) Q6H 15 kg (33 lb) = 1½ tsp (7.5 mL) Q6H 20 kg (44 lb) = 2 tsp (10 mL) Q6H	**Food:** Take 1 hour before or 2 hours after meals. **Important side effects:** Bad taste, GI upset.

(continued)

Drug, Its Forms and Dosage Increments	Children and Adult Dosages and Instructions	Information and Important Side Effects
	40 kg (88 lb) = Use adult dose **Adult:** 250-500 mg PO four times daily for 10-14 days.	

EARS – Otitis Externa, Malignant (*Pseudomonas aeruginosa*)

Comment: Consider urgent ENT, infectious disease consult. Only early, very mild cases appropriate for outpatient therapy. Assess need for IV antibiotics. Usually occurs in diabetic patients.

Drug, Its Forms and Dosage Increments	Children and Adult Dosages and Instructions	Information and Important Side Effects
Ciprofloxacin* (Cipro®) Pregnancy: C; Lactation: Unsafe **Tabs:** 250 mg, 500 mg, 750 mg - $$$$ - >$$$$	**Adult:** 750 mg PO twice daily for 7-14 days.	**Food:** Take 1 hour before or 2 hours after a meal. May take with food if it causes GI upset. Make take 2 hours before or 6 hours after sucralfate, antacids, aluminum, magnesium, calcium, zinc, iron, vitamins, or mineral supplements. **Important side effects:** Photosensitivity, dizziness. **Reduce dose in renal disease (CrCl <50 mL/min).**
Levofloxacin* (Levaquin®) Pregnancy: C; Lactation: Unsafe **Tabs:** 250 mg, 500 mg - $$$ - >$$$$	**Adult:** 500 mg PO once daily for 7-14 days.	**Food:** Do not take within 2 hours of antacids, magnesium, calcium, zinc, iron, aluminum, sucralfate, vitamins, or mineral supplements. **Important side effects:** Photosensitivity, dizziness. **Reduce dose in renal disease (CrCl <50 mL/min).**

Drug	Dosage	Comments
Imipenem/cilastatin IV (Primaxin®) Pregnancy: C; Lactation: Unk **OR** Other IV drug with good antipseudomonal coverage. Examples include ciprofloxacin, ceftazidime, or a combination of an aminoglycoside and piperacillin.	**Adult:** 500 mg IV every 6 hours. 7-14 days (or until switch to alternate oral agent is appropriate).	**Important side effects:** Confusion, seizures.

EARS – Otitis Externa, Otomycosis (Fungal)

Drug	Dosage	Comments
Nystatin* (Mycostatin®, Nilstat®) Generics available Pregnancy: B; Lactation: Safe **Cream 100,000 U/g:** 15 g, 30 g - <$ **Oint 100,000 U/g:** 15 g, 30 g - <$	**Children and Adult:** Apply topically with swab twice daily for 10 days.	**Important side effects:** Well tolerated. **Prevention:** 1:1 mixture of rubbing alcohol and vinegar in external canal after swimming.
Clotrimazole Sol* (Lotrimin®) Pregnancy: B; Lactation: Unk **Topical Solution 1%:** 10 mL - <$	**Children and Adult:** Instill 2-4 drops in the affected ear(s) twice daily for 7 days.	**Important side effects:** May cause local irritation. **Caution:** Use only with intact tympanic membrane.
Acetic acid 2%* (VoSol® otic) Pregnancy: Unk; Lactation: Unk **Sol 2%:** 15-mL bottle - <$	**Children and Adult:** Saturate cotton wick and insert in ear. Apply 3-5 drops to wick every 4-6 hours for 24 hours. Remove wick, then instill 3-5 drops in affected ear(s) three to four times daily for as long as needed.	

(continued)

Drug, Its Forms and Dosage Increments	Children and Adult Dosages and Instructions	Information and Important Side Effects
EARS – Otitis Media (*Streptococcus pneumoniae, Haemophilus influenzae, Moraxella catarrhalis*) **Note:** In one third of cases no bacterial pathogen is identified. Benefits of antibiotic therapy in question. (**AOM Tx Duration:** If <2 years × 10 days. If ≥2 years × 5-7 days. See *Pediatr Infect Dis J* 1999;18:1–9.)		
Amoxicillin - Drug of choice, especially if no antibiotics used in previous 30 days. If clinical failure on day 3, use alternative beta-lactam listed. (Amoxil®, Trimox®) Generics available Pregnancy: B; Lactation: Safe **Caps:** 250 mg, 500 mg - <\$ **Tabs:** 500 mg, 875 mg - <\$ **Chewable Tabs:** 125 mg, 250 mg **Oral Susp:** 50 mg/mL, 125 mg/5 mL, 250 mg/5 mL - <\$ - \$	**Children: Dosing:** 40-90 mg/kg/day (max 1500 mg/day) in divided doses three times daily. If <2 years × 10 days. If ≥2 years × 5-7 days. **125 mg/5 mL at 40 mg/kg/day or 250 mg/5 mL at 80 mg/kg/day** 8 kg (18 lb) = 1 tsp (5 mL) Q8H 13 kg (29 lb) = 1½ tsp (7.5 mL) Q8H 17 kg (37 lb) = 2 tsp (10 mL) Q8H 21 kg (46 lb) = 2½ tsp (12.5 mL) (NTE 500 mg) Q8H 25 kg (55 lb) = 3 tsp (15 mL) (NTE 500 mg) Q8H **Adult:** 875 mg twice daily **or** 500 mg three times daily for 5-10 days.	**Food:** May take with or without meals. **Important side effects:** Diarrhea and nausea. May cause nonallergic maculopapular rash. **Reduce dose in renal disease (CrCl <30 mL/min).**
Amoxicillin/clavulanate (Augmentin®) Pregnancy: B; Lactation: Unk **Q12H Formulations (7:1):** **Tabs:** 875 mg/125 mg	**Children:** 80-90 mg amoxicillin component/kg/day (max 1600 mg/day) in divided doses two times daily. If <2 years × 10 days. If ≥2 years × 5-7 days. 14:1 (ES-600) formulation is advised,	**Food:** Take with food to reduce diarrhea. **Important side effects:** Diarrhea (common), nausea, rash. May cause nonallergic maculopapular rash.

Chewable Tabs:
200 mg/28.5 mg, 400 mg/57 mg
Oral Susp:
200 mg/28.5 mg/5 mL,
400 mg/57 mg/5 mL
Augmentin ES-600 Powder for Oral Suspension (14:1): 600 mg/42.9 mg/5 mL
Cost of 10-day course:
Child - $$$ Adult - >$$$$
Note: Q12H dosing may improve compliance compared to Q8H dosing.

especially if antibiotic exposure for otitis media in preceding 3 months and either age ≤2 years or daycare attendance. If low likelihood of resistant *S. pneumoniae*, may use 7:1 formulation; however, limit clavulanate to no more than 10 mg/kg/day (amoxicillin 70 mg/kg/day).

Q12H using 600/5 mL susp @ 90 mg/kg/day
8 kg (18 lb) = 3 mL Q12H
12 kg (26 lb) = 4.5 mL Q12H
16 kg (35 lb) = 6 mL Q12H
20 kg (44 lb) = 7.5 mL Q12H
24 kg (53 lb) = 9.0 mL Q12H
28 kg (62 lb) = 10.5 mL Q12H
32 kg (70 lb) = 12.0 mL Q12H
36 kg (79 lb) = 13.5 mL Q12H
>40 kg = Experience not available.

If low likelihood of resistant *S. pneumoniae*, may use 7:1 formulation; however, limit clavulanate to no more than 10 mg/kg/day (amoxicillin 70 mg/kg/day).

Q12H using 400 mg/57 mg/5 mL suspension @ 70 mg/kg/day:
11 kg (24 lb) = 1 tsp (5 mL) Q12H
17 kg (37 lb) = 1½ (7.5 mL) tsp Q12H
23 kg (51 lb) = 2 tsp (10 mL) Q12H
>23 kg = Use adult dose.

Adult: 500-875 mg twice daily for 10 days.

Use with caution in hepatic disease. Reduce dose if renal impairment (CrCl <30 mL/min).

(continued)

Drug, Its Forms and Dosage Increments	Children and Adult Dosages and Instructions	Information and Important Side Effects
Cefpodoxime (Vantin®) Pregnancy: B; Lactation: Unsafe **Tabs:** 100 mg, 200 mg **Oral Susp:** 50 mg/5 mL, 100 mg/5 mL 50 mg/5 mL Q12H × 10 days - $$ 200 mg PO Q12H × 5 days - $$	**Children >2 months to 12 years:** 10 mg/kg/day (NTE 400 mg) in divided doses once or twice daily. If <2 years × 10 days. If ≥2 years × 5-7 days. **100 mg/5 mL @ 10 mg/kg/day** 10 kg (22 lb) = 1 tsp (5 mL) Q24H 20 kg (44 lb) = 2 tsp (10 mL) Q24H 30 kg (66 lb) = 3 tsp Q24H **Adult:** 100-200 mg PO twice daily for 5-7 days.	**Food:** Take tablets with food. Suspension may be taken without regard to food. **Important side effects:** Diarrhea.
Cefuroxime axetil (Ceftin®) Pregnancy: B; Lactation: Unsafe **Tabs:** 125 mg, 250 mg, 500 mg **Oral Susp:** 125 mg/5 mL, 250 mg/5 mL 125 mg/5 mL Q12H × 10 days - $$ 250 mg PO Q12H × 5 days - $$	**Children >3 months to 12 years:** 30 mg/kg/day (NTE 1,000 mg/day) in divided doses twice daily. If <2 years × 10 days. If ≥2 years × 5-7 days. **125 mg/5 mL @ 30 mg/kg/day** 8 kg (18 lb) = 1 tsp (5 mL) Q12H 12.5 kg (27 lb) = 1½ tsp (7.5 mL) Q12H 17 kg (37 lb) = 2 tsp (10 mL) Q12H 25 kg (55 lb) = 1 tbsp Q12H 33 kg (73 lb) = Use adult dose. **Adult:** 250-500 mg PO twice daily for 5-7 days.	**Food:** Take suspension with food. Tablets may be taken without regard to food. **Important side effects:** Nausea, vomiting, diarrhea.
Trimethoprim/Sulfamethoxazole* **Alternative for beta-lactam intolerance.** (Bactrim®, Septra®)	**Children >2 months:** 8-10 mg/kg/day TMP component (max 320 mg/day) in divided doses twice daily for 5-10 days.	**Food:** May take without regard to food. Encourage fluids.

Generics available Pregnancy: C; Lactation: Unsafe **Single Strength (SS) Tabs:** 80 mg/400 mg **Double Strength (DS) Tabs:** 160 mg/800 mg **Oral Susp:** 40 mg/200 mg per 5 mL 10 mL Q12H × 10 days <$ - $ DS Tab PO Q12H × 10 days - $ May be less active against penicillin resistant *S. pneumoniae.*	**8-10 mg/kg/day @ 40 mg/200 mg/5 mL** 10 kg (22 lb) = 1 tsp (5 mL) Q12H 20 kg (44 lb) = 2 tsp (10 mL) or 1 SS tab Q12H 30 kg (66 lb) = 3 tsp (15 mL) or 1½ SS tab Q12H 40 kg (88 lb) = 4 tsp (20 mL) or 2 SS tabs or 1 DS tab Q12H **Adult:** 1 DS tab PO twice daily for 5-10 days.	**Important side effects:** Photosensitivity, rash.

EARS – Otitis Media – Failed Treatment

Levofloxacin* (Levaquin®) Pregnancy: C; Lactation: Unsafe **Tabs:** 250 mg, 500 mg - >$$$$	**Adult:** 500 mg PO once daily for 10-14 days.	**Food:** With or without meals. Do not take within 2 hours of antacids, magnesium, calcium supplements, zinc, aluminum, sucralfate, vitamins, or minerals (iron or zinc). **Important side effects:** Photosensitivity, dizziness. **Reduce dose if renal impairment (CrCl <50 mL/min).**
Ceftriaxone (Rocephin®) Pregnancy: B; Lactation: Unk **Vials:** 250 mg, 500 mg, 1,000 mg 1 g - $$$	**Children and Adult:** 50 mg/kg (max 1 g) IM daily × 1-3 days.	

(continued)

Drug, Its Forms and Dosage Increments	Children and Adult Dosages and Instructions	Information and Important Side Effects
EARS – Mastoiditis, Simple (*Streptococcus pneumoniae, Streptococcus pyogenes, Staphylococcus aureus*) **Comment:** Empirical treatment same as acute otitis media. May need to adjust therapy if cultures show *S. aureus* or gram-negative enteric bacilli.		
Amoxicillin/clavulanate (Augmentin®) Pregnancy: B; Lactation: Unk **Q12H Formulations:** **Tabs:** 500 mg/125 mg, 875 mg/125 mg **Chewable Tabs:** 400 mg/57 mg **Oral Susp:** 400 mg/57 mg/5 mL, 600 mg/42.9 mg/5 mL Child - $$$ Adult - >$$$$	**Children:** 80-90 mg amoxicillin component/kg/day (max 1600 mg/day) in divided doses two or three times daily. If <2 years × 10 days. If ≥2 years × 5-7 days. **Q12H using 400 mg/5 mL susp @ 90 mg/kg/day** 10 kg (22 lb) = 1 tsp (5 mL) Q12H 15 kg (33 lb) = 1½ tsp (7.5 mL) Q12H 20 kg (44 lb) = 2 tsp (10 mL) Q12H >20 kg = Use adult dose. **Q12H using 600 mg/5 mL susp @ 90 mg/kg/day** 8 kg (18 lb) = 3 mL Q12H 12 kg (26 lb) = 4.5 mL Q12H 16 kg (35 lb) = 6 mL Q12H 20 kg (44 lb) = 7.5 mL Q12H 24 kg (53 lb) = 9.0 mL Q12H 28 kg (62 lb) = 10.5 mL Q12H 32 kg (70 lb) = 12.0 mL Q12H 36 kg (79 lb) = 13.5 mL Q12H >40 kg = Experience not available. **Adult:** 500-875 mg twice daily for 10 days.	**Food:** Take with food to reduce diarrhea. **Important side effects:** Diarrhea (common), nausea, rash. May cause nonallergic maculopapular rash.

	Note: Q12H dosing may improve compliance compared to Q8H dosing.	
Cefuroxime axetil (Ceftin®) Pregnancy: B; Lactation: Unsafe **Tabs:** 125 mg, 250 mg, 500 mg **Oral Suspension:** 125 mg/5 mL, 250 mg/5 mL 125 mg/5 mL Q12H × 10 days - $$ 250 mg PO Q12H × 5 days - $$	**Children >3 months to 12 years:** 30 mg/kg/day (NTE 1,000 mg/day) in divided doses twice daily × 10 days. **125 mg/5 mL @ 30 mg/kg/day** 8 kg (18 lb) = 1 tsp (5 mL) Q12H 12.5 kg (27 lb) = 1½ tsp (7.5 mL) Q12H 17 kg (37 lb) = 2 tsp (10 mL) Q12H 25 kg (55 lb) = 3 tsp (15 mL) Q12H 33 kg (73 lb) = Use adult dose. **Adult:** 250-500 mg PO twice daily for 10 days.	**Food:** Take suspension with food, tablets without regard to food.

EARS – Mastoiditis, Malignant (*Streptococcus pneumoniae*, *Streptococcus pyogenes*, *Staphylococcus aureus*)

Comment: Requires parenteral antimicrobial therapy. If hospitalization is delayed, initiate empiric therapy with ceftriaxone IM, an oral fluoroquinolone, or other therapy appropriate for acute otitis media.

FACE – Acne Rosacea – Mild or Suppressive (Unknown cause)

Metronidazole Gel* MetroGel® Pregnancy: B; Lactation: Unsafe **Topical Gel 0.75%**	**Children:** Should not need until adolescence. **Adult:** Apply twice daily. (Use sparingly.)

(continued)

FACE – Acne Rosacea – Mild or Suppressive (Unknown cause)

Drug, Its Forms and Dosage Increments	Children and Adult Dosages and Instructions	Information and Important Side Effects
Clindamycin Topical* Cleocin T® Pregnancy: B; Lactation: Unsafe **Topical Gel 1%:** 7.5 g, 30 g **Lotion 1%:** 60 mL	**Children:** Should not need until adolescence. **Adult:** Apply twice daily. (Use sparingly).	
Erythromycin Gel* Erygel®, EryDerm® Pregnancy: B; Lactation: Unsafe **Topical Gel 2%**	**Children:** Should not need until adolescence. **Adult:** Apply twice daily. (Use sparingly).	

FACE – Acne Rosacea – Moderate to Severe (Unknown cause)

Drug, Its Forms and Dosage Increments	Children and Adult Dosages and Instructions	Information and Important Side Effects
Doxycycline* (Vibramycin®) Generics available Pregnancy: D; Lactation: Unsafe **Caps:** 50 mg, 100 mg **Tabs:** 100 mg	**Children:** Should not need until adolescence. **Adult:** 100 mg PO twice daily.	**Food:** May take with food if GI upset occurs. Take 1 hour before or 2 hours after antacids, iron, milk, or other dairy products. Take with full glass of water to prevent esophagitis. **Important side effects:** Photosensitivity (use sunscreen), esophagitis. May discolor fingernails.
Tetracycline* (Sumycin®, Achromycin V®) Generics available Pregnancy: D; Lactation: Unsafe	**Adult:** 250 mg PO four times daily for 7-10 days, then taper to 250-500 mg PO daily.	**Food:** Take 1 hour before or 2 hours after meals. Take with full glass of water to minimize esophagitis. Do not take within three hours of antacids,

Caps: 250 mg, 500 mg **Tabs:** 250 mg, 500 mg		iron, milk, or other dairy or calcium products. **Important side effects:** Photosensitivity (use sunscreen), esophagitis. May discolor fingernails. Rash, nausea, vomiting, diarrhea, superinfection, hepatitis, renal damage.

FACE – Acne Rosacea – Resistant

Trimethoprim/Sulfamethoxazole* (Bactrim®, Septra®) Generics available Pregnancy: C; Lactation: Unsafe **Single Strength (SS) Tabs:** 80 mg/400 mg **Double Strength (DS) Tabs:** 160 mg/800 mg <$ - $	**Adult:** 1 DS tablet PO twice daily for 10-21 days.	**Food:** May take without regard to food. Encourage fluids. **Important side effects:** Photosensitivity, rash. **Reduce dose if renal impairment (CrCl <30 mL/min).**

FACE – Acne Vulgaris – Mild, Noninflammatory – Comedolytic

Adapalene (Differin®) Pregnancy: C; Lactation: Unknown **Gel 0.1%:** 15 g, 45 g	**Adolescent and Adult:** Apply once daily at bedtime after cleansing the area to be treated. Cover entire affected area lightly. Wash hands after use. Exacerbation of condition may be seen early in therapy but, unless severe, is not a reason to	**Caution:** Keep away from eye(s), mouth, angles of nose, and mucous membranes. Avoid excessive exposure to sun and sunlamps. Do not apply over sunburned skin. Avoid coadministering with topical products,

(continued)

Drug, Its Forms and Dosage Increments	Children and Adult Dosages and Instructions	Information and Important Side Effects
	discontinue. Therapeutic results should be seen after 8-12 weeks of therapy.	which may cause irritation to the skin. This includes products containing sulfur, resorcinol, benzoyl peroxide, or salicylic acid. **Important side effects:** May cause irritation, burning, and stinging on application. Erythema, scaling, dryness, and other local irritation may occur, especially during the first few weeks of therapy. Unless irritation is severe, application should continue and irritation usually lessens with continued use. If excessive irritation occurs, application should be discontinued or applied less frequently.
Azelaic Acid Azelex® Pregnancy: B; Lactation: Caution **Cream 20%:** 30 g - $$	**Adolescent and Adult:** Thoroughly massage in to affected area twice daily after washing, and pat dry. Improvement usually seen within 4 weeks. Wash hands after application.	**Important side effects:** May rarely cause hypopigmentation; monitor closely in dark-skinned persons. May cause skin irritation. Avoid contact with eye(s).
Benzoyl Peroxide 5-10% Many brands OTC Pregnancy: C; Lactation: Unk **Cream 5% and 10%** **Gel 2.5%, 5%, 10%, and 20%**	**Adolescent and Adult:** Begin with a low-potency strength and increase strength and frequency as tolerated. Apply to skin (after cleansing) up to 1-3 times daily.	**Caution:** Do not apply to inflamed or raw skin, mucous membranes, eye(s), eyelids, or lips. May bleach colored fabrics.

5% 60 mL - $16.50
Liquid 2.5%, 5%, and 10%
5% 120 mL - $15.75
Lotion 5%, 5.5%, 10%

***Note: Gels may be more potent, longer lasting, and more irritating than creams or lotions.**

Important side effects: May cause stinging, drying, or peeling of the skin. Irritation may be reduced by applying to dry skin 30 minutes after washing. Discontinue if irritation is excessive.

Tretinoin (trans-retinoic acid) Topical
(Retin-A®, Avita®)
Pregnancy: C; Lactation: Unknown
Cream: 0.0025%, 0.05%, 0.1%: 20 g, 40 g
Gel 0.025%, 0.01%: 15 g, 45 g
Liquid 0.05%: 28 mL

Adolescent and Adult: Apply once daily at bedtime after cleansing the area to be treated. Cover entire affected area lightly. Wash hands after use. Improvement may be seen in 2-3 weeks, but may not be optimal until after 6 weeks.

Caution: Keep away from eye(s), mouth, angles of nose, and mucous membranes. Avoid excessive exposure to sun and sunlamps. Do not apply over sunburned skin. Avoid coadministering with topical products containing sulfur, resorcinol, benzoyl peroxide, or salicylic acid.
Important side effects: Application may cause transient sensation of warmth or stinging. Excessive application may cause irritation or peeling of skin. If excessive redness, burning, or peeling occurs, reduce frequency of use or temporarily discontinue or reduce strength of product.

FACE – Acne Vulgaris – Mild, Inflammatory (*Propionibacterium acnes*) - Comedolytic + Topical or Oral Antibiotic

Erythromycin Topical*
(Erygel®, EryDerm®, Staticin®)
Generics available

Children: Should not need until adolescence.

Important side effects: Local irritation and dryness.

(continued)

Drug, Its Forms and Dosage Increments	Children and Adult Dosages and Instructions	Information and Important Side Effects
Pregnancy: B, C; Lactation: Unsafe **Gel 2%:** 30 g - $$ **Solution 1½% & 2%:** 60 mL - <$ **Pledgets 2%**	**Adolescent and Adult:** Apply twice daily after cleansing. May see response in 3-8 weeks; however, may require 12 weeks for full response. Continue as long as satisfactory response is maintained and side effects do not occur.	
Clindamycin Topical* (Cleocin T®) Pregnancy: B; Lactation: Safe **Gel 1%:** 30 g - $$ **Sol 1%:** 30 mL - $ **Lotion 1%:** 60 mL - $$$	**Children:** Should not need until adolescence. **Adolescent and Adult:** Apply Q12H after cleansing. May see improvement in 2-6 weeks; however, may require 12 weeks for full response. Continue as long as satisfactory response is maintained and significant side effects do not occur.	**Important side effects:** Local irritation and dryness. May rarely cause diarrhea.
Doxycycline* (Vibramycin®) Generics available Pregnancy: D; Lactation: Unsafe **Caps:** 50 mg, 100 mg <$/month **Tabs:** 50 mg, 100 mg	**Adolescent and Adult:** 50-100 mg PO twice daily.	**Food:** May take with food if GI upset occurs. Take 1 hour before or 2 hours after antacids, iron, milk, or other dairy products. Take with full glass of water to prevent esophagitis. **Important side effects:** Photosensitivity (use sunscreen), esophagitis. May discolor fingernails.
Erythromycin Base* (E-Mycin®)	**Adolescent and Adult:** 250 mg PO four times daily or 500 mg PO twice daily. If no	**Food:** May take with or without meals. Take with food if GI upset occurs.

Generics available Pregnancy: B; Lactation: Unsafe **Tabs:** 250 mg, 500 mg $/month for maintenance	response in 2-3 weeks or severe acne: 500 mg PO four times daily. Maintenance dose: 250-500 mg once daily.	**Important side effects:** GI upset, hepatitis.
Tetracycline* (Sumycin®, Tetracap®) Generics available Pregnancy: D; Lactation: Unsafe **Caps:** 250 mg, 500 mg <$/month **Tabs:** 250 mg, 500 mg	**Adolescent and Adult:** 250 mg PO four times daily for 2-3 weeks, then taper to 250-500 mg once daily. If no response after 2-3 weeks, increase to 500 mg PO four times daily before tapering.	**Food:** Take 1 hour before or 2 hours after meals. Take with full glass of water to minimize esophagitis. Do not take within 3 hours of antacids, iron, milk, or other dairy or calcium products. **Important side effects:** Photosensitivity (use sunscreen), esophagitis. May discolor fingernails. Rash, nausea, vomiting, diarrhea, superinfection, hepatitis, renal damage.
Minocycline* (Minocin®) Pregnancy: D; Lactation: Unsafe **Caps:** 50 mg, 100 mg	**Adolescent and Adult:** 100 mg PO twice daily. *Costs ($100/mo) and has more side effects than tetracycline or doxycycline.*	**Food:** Take with full glass of water to prevent esophagitis. Do not take with dairy products, antacids, calcium, zinc, or iron products. **Important side effects:** GI upset, esophagitis, photosensitivity, drowsiness, dizziness, discoloration of skin.

FACE – Acne Vulgaris – Inflammatory (*Propionibacterium acnes*) See drugs listed in previous section.
Use in combination.
Comedolytic + Topical antibiotic + Oral antibiotic

(continued)

Drug, Its Forms and Dosage Increments	Children and Adult Dosages and Instructions	Information and Important Side Effects
FACE – Acne Vulgaris – Severe (*Propionibacterium acnes*) Less than 50% response to three-agent therapy after 5-6 months.		
Isotretinoin (Accutane®) **Pregnancy: D; Lactation:** Unsafe **Caps:** 10 mg, 20 mg, 40 mg **Prescribers of isotretinoin should be completely familiar with the risks associated with its use. The information provided here is brief and not intended to familiarize the prescriber with all risks involved. Prescriptions are limited to a 1-month supply with no automatic refill. Patient and prescriber must sign consent form from manufacturer.**	**Adolescent and Adult:** 0.5-1 mg/kg/day in 2 divided doses for 15-20 weeks or until the total cyst count is decreased by 70%, whichever occurs first. When disease is very severe with scarring or is primarily manifested on the trunk, patient may require dose adjustments up to 2 mg/kg/day as tolerated.	**Food:** Isotretinoin should be taken with food, which significantly increases absorption. Before upward dose adjustments are made, patients should be questioned about their compliance with food instructions. Take with full glass of water to prevent esophagitis. **Major side effects:** Known to cause major fetal abnormalities. Verify pregnancy status of female patients and educate them on effective contraception. Do not use in women of childbearing potential not capable of following an effective contraceptive program. May cause CNS side effects, including psychosis or depression. May cause pseudotumor cerebri. Use with tetracycline may increase risk. Do not administer with tetracycline or vitamin A. **Other side effects:** Photosensitivity, pruritus, insomnia, hyperglycemia,

		hypertriglyceridemia, decreased night vision, intolerance to contact lenses, others.

FACE – Sinusitis – Acute, Mild to Moderate (*Streptococcus pneumoniae*, *Haemophilus influenzae*, *Moraxella catarrhalis*)

Amoxicillin (Amoxil®) Pregnancy: B; Lactation: Unk **Caps:** 250 mg, 500 mg **Tabs:** 500 mg, 875 mg **Chewable Tabs:** 125 mg, 250 mg **Susp:** 125 mg/5 mL, 250 mg/5 mL, 400 mg/5 mL **Oral drops:** 50 mg/mL <$	**Children:** 45-90 mg/kg/day (max 1500 mg/day) in divided doses three times daily for 10-14 days. **250 mg/5 mL at 90 mg/kg/day** 8 kg (18 lb) = 1 tsp (5 mL) Q8H 17 kg (37 lb) = 2 tsp (10 mL) Q8H >17 kg = Use adult dose. **Adult:** 500 mg PO three times daily for 10-14 days.	**Food:** May take with or without meals. **Important side effects:** Diarrhea and nausea. May cause nonallergic maculopapular rash. **Reduce dose if renal impairment (CrCl <30 mL/min).**
Amoxicillin/clavulanate (Augmentin®) Pregnancy: B; Lactation: Unk **Q12H Formulations:** **Tabs:** 500 mg/125 mg, 875 mg/125 mg **Oral Susp:** 200 mg/28.5 mg/5 mL, 400 mg/57 mg/5 mL **Chewable Tab:** 200 mg/28.5 mg, 400 mg/57 mg **Q8H Formulations:** **Tabs:** 250 mg/125 mg, 500 mg/125 mg	**Neonates and infants <3 months:** **Use 125 mg/31.25 mg/5 mL suspension.** 30 mg/kg/day in divided doses every 12 hours **Children ≥3 months up to 40 kg:** 40-45 mg amoxicillin component/kg/day (max 1600 mg/day) in divided doses two or three times daily for 10-14 days. **Q12H using 200 mg/5 mL susp @ 45 mg/kg/day** 9 kg (20 lb) = 1 tsp (5 mL) Q12H	**Food:** Take with food to reduce diarrhea. **Important side effects:** Diarrhea (common), nausea, rash. May cause nonallergic maculopapular rash. **Use with caution in hepatic disease.** **Reduce dose in renal impairment (CrCl <30 mL/min).**

(continued)

Drug, Its Forms and Dosage Increments	Children and Adult Dosages and Instructions	Information and Important Side Effects
Oral Susp: 125 mg/31.25 mg/5 mL, 250 mg/62.5 mg/5 mL **Chewable Tab:** 125 mg/31.25 mg, 250 mg/62.5 mg Child - $$$ Adult - >$$$$	13 kg (29 lb) = 1½ tsp (7.5 mL) Q12H 18 kg (40 lb) = 2 tsp (10 mL) Q12H **Q12H using 400 mg/5 mL susp @ 45 mg/kg/day** 18 kg (40 lb) = 1 tsp (5 mL) Q12H 27 kg (59 lb) = 1½ tsp (7.5 mL) Q12H 35 kg (77 lb) = 2 tsp (10 mL) Q12H >40 kg = Use adult dosing (max 875 mg Q12H). **Adult:** 500-875 mg twice daily for 10-14 days. Note: Q12H dosing may improve compliance compared to Q8H dosing.	
Cefpodoxime (Vantin®) Pregnancy: B; Lactation: Unsafe **Tabs:** 100 mg, 200 mg **Oral Susp:** 50 mg/5 mL, 100 mg/5 mL 50 mg/5 mL Q12H × 10 days - $$ 200 mg PO Q12H × 10 days - $$$$	**Children >5 months to 12 years:** 10 mg/kg/day (max 400 mg) in divided doses twice daily for 10 days. **100 mg/5 mL @ 10 mg/kg/day** 10 kg (22 lb) = 1 tsp (5 mL) Q24H 20 kg (44 lb) = 2 tsp (10 mL) Q24H 30 kg (66 lb) = 3 tsp Q24H **12 years to Adult:** 200-400 mg twice daily for 10-14 days.	**Food:** Take tablet with food. Suspension may be taken without regard to food. **Important side effects:** Diarrhea.
Cefuroxime axetil (Ceftin®) Pregnancy: B; Lactation: Unsafe	**Children >3 months to 12 years:** 30 mg/kg/day (max 1,000 mg/day) in divided doses twice daily for 10 days.	**Food:** Take suspension with food. Tablets may be taken without regard to food.

Tabs: 125 mg, 250 mg, 500 mg **Oral Suspension:** 125 mg/5 mL, 250 mg/5 mL 125 mg/5 mL Q12H × 10 days - $$ 250 mg PO Q12H × 10 days - $$$$	**125 mg/5 mL @ 30 mg/kg/day** 8 kg (18 lb) = 1 tsp (5 mL) Q12H 12.5 kg (27 lb) = 1½ tsp (7.5 mL) Q12H 17 kg (37 lb) = 2 tsp (10 mL) Q12H 25 kg (55 lb) = 3 tsp (15 mL) Q12H 33 kg (73 lb) = Use adult dose. **12 years to Adults:** 250-500 mg PO twice daily for 7-14 days.	**Important side effects:** Nausea, vomiting, diarrhea.

FACE – Sinusitis – Acute, Mild to Moderate with Beta-lactam Allergy (*Streptococcus pneumoniae, Haemophilus influenzae, Moraxella catarrhalis*)

Azithromycin* (Zithromax®) Pregnancy: B; Lactation: Unk **Tabs:** 250 mg and Z-Pak (500 mg × 1 day, then 250 mg daily × 4) **Oral Suspension:** 100 mg/5 mL, 200 mg/5 mL 20-kg child - $$ Z-Pak - $$$	**Children ≥6 months:** 10 mg/kg/day (max 500 mg) daily × 1 day, then 5 mg/kg/day (max 250 mg) daily × 4 days. **100 mg/5 mL** 10 kg (22 lb) = 1 tsp (5 mL)/day × 1 day, then ½ tsp (2.5 mL) daily for days 2-5. **200 mg/5 mL** 20 kg (44 lb) = 1 tsp (5 mL)/day × 1 day, then ½ tsp (2.5 mL) daily for days 2-5. 30 kg (66 lb) = 1.5 tsp/day × 1 day, then ¾ tsp daily for days 2-5. **Adult:** Dispense one Z-Pak.	**Food:** Suspension, 1 hour before or 2 hours after food. Tablets, without regard to food. **Important side effects:** Nausea, diarrhea, elevated LFTs.
Clarithromycin* (Biaxin®, Biaxin XL®) Pregnancy: C; Lactation: Unk	**Children ≥6 months:** 15 mg/kg/day (max 1,000 mg/day) in divided doses twice daily for 10-14 days.	**Food:** Extended release tablet with food. Others without regard to food. **Important side effects:** Nausea.

(continued)

Drug, Its Forms and Dosage Increments	Children and Adult Dosages and Instructions	Information and Important Side Effects
Tabs: 250 mg, 500 mg **Extended Release Tab (XL):** 500 mg **Oral Susp:** 125 mg/5 mL, 250 mg/5 mL 250 mg/5 mL Q12H × 10 days - $$$ 500 mg PO Q12H × 10 days - $$$$	**125 mg/5 mL @ 15 mg/kg/day** 9 kg (20 lb) = ½ tsp (2.5 mL) Q12H 17 kg (37 lb) = 1 tsp (5 mL) Q12H **250 mg/5 mL @ 15 mg/kg/day** 17 kg (37 lb) = ½ tsp (2.5 mL) Q12H 25 kg (55 lb) = ¾ tsp Q12H 33 kg (73 lb) = 1 tsp (5 mL) Q12H **Adult:** 500 mg PO twice daily or 1 g XL PO once daily for 10-14 days.	
Erythromycin estolate or base* (Ilosone®, E-mycin®, Ery-Tab®) Generics available Pregnancy: B; Lactation: Unsafe **Estolate:** **Tabs:** 500 mg **Caps:** 250 mg **Oral Susp:** 125 mg/5 mL, 250 mg/5 mL 250 mg/5 mL Q12H × 10 days - $ **Base:** **Tabs:** 250 mg, 333 mg, 500 mg **Caps:** 250 mg 500 mg PO Q6H × 10 days - $	**Children:** 20-40 mg/kg/day estolate (max 2 g/day) in two to four divided doses daily for 10-14 days. **125 mg/5 mL @ 20 mg/kg/day** 4-6 kg (10-15 lb) = ½ tsp (2.5 mL) Q12H 7-11 kg (16-25 lb) = 1 tsp (5 mL) Q12H 12-16 kg (26-35 lb) = 1½ tsp (7.5 mL) Q12H **250 mg/5 mL @ 20 mg/kg/day** 17-25 kg (37-55 lb) = 1 tsp (5 mL) Q12H 26-37 kg (57-81 lb) = 1½ tsp (7.5 mL) Q12H >38 kg (83 lb) = 500 mg Q12H **Adult:** Erythromycin base or estolate 500 mg PO four times daily for 10-14 days.	**Food:** May take with or without meals. Take with food if causes GI upset. **Important side effects:** GI upset, hepatitis.

Drug	Dosage	Comments
Trimethoprim/Sulfamethoxazole* (Bactrim®, Septra®) Generics available Pregnancy: C; Lactation: Unsafe **Single Strength (SS) Tabs:** 80 mg/400 mg **Double Strength (DS) Tabs:** 160 mg/800 mg **Oral Susp:** 40 mg/200 mg per 5 mL 10 mL Q12H × 10 days <$ DS Tab PO Q12H × 10 days - $	**Children >2 months:** 8-10 mg/kg/day TMP component (max 320 mg/day) in divided doses twice daily for 10-14 days. **8-10 mg/kg/day @ 40 mg/200 mg/5 mL** 10 kg (22 lb) = 1 tsp (5 mL) Q12H 20 kg (44 lb) = 2 tsp (10 mL) or 1 SS Tab Q12H 30 kg (66 lb) = 3 tsp (15 mL) or 1½ SS Tab Q12H 40 kg (88 lb) = 4 tsp (20 mL) or 2 SS Tabs or 1 DS Tab Q12H **Adult:** 1 DS Tab PO twice daily for 10-14 days.	**Food:** May take without regard to food. Encourage fluids. **Important side effects:** Photosensitivity, rash. **Reduce dose if renal impairment (CrCl <30 mL/min).**

FACE – Sinusitis – Acute – Failed Therapy or Antibiotic Use in the Past 4-6 Weeks (*Streptococcus pneumoniae, Haemophilus influenzae, Moraxella catarrhalis*)

Drug	Dosage	Comments
Gatifloxacin* (Tequin®) Pregnancy: C; Lactation: Unsafe Tabs: 400 mg - $$$$	**Adult:** 400 mg PO Q24H for 10 days.	**Food:** May take with or without meals. Do not take within 4 hours of sucralfate, antacids, vitamins or mineral products. **Important side effects:** Dizziness, photosensitivity, headache. **Reduce dose if renal impairment (CrCl <40 mL/min).**
Levofloxacin* (Levaquin®)	**Adult:** 500 mg PO once daily for 10-14 days.	**Food:** May take with or without meals. Do not take within 2 hours of antacids,

(continued)

Drug, Its Forms and Dosage Increments	Children and Adult Dosages and Instructions	Information and Important Side Effects
Pregnancy: C; Lactation: Unsafe **Tabs:** 250 mg, 500 mg - $$$$		magnesium, calcium supplements, zinc, aluminum, sucralfate, vitamins, or minerals (iron or zinc). **Important side effects:** Photosensitivity, dizziness. **Reduce dose if renal impairment (CrCl <50 mL/min).**
Moxifloxacin* (Avelox®) Pregnancy: C; Lactation: Unk **Tabs:** 400 mg - >$$$$	**Adult:** 400 mg PO once daily for 10 days.	**Food:** May take without regard to food. Must take 4 hours before or 8 hours after sucralfate, antacids, aluminum, magnesium, calcium, zinc, iron, vitamins, or mineral supplements. **Important side effects:** Photosensitivity, dizziness, headache, insomnia, rash (may be severe), drug interactions.

PHARYNX / NECK – Tonsillitis/Pharyngitis by Pathogen (Group A *Streptococcus*)

Drug, Its Forms and Dosage Increments	Children and Adult Dosages and Instructions	Information and Important Side Effects
Penicillin V Potassium (Pen Vee K®) Generics Available Pregnancy: B; Lactation: Unk **Tabs:** 250 mg, 500 mg **Oral Susp:** 125 mg/5 mL, 250 mg/5 mL	**Children <12 years:** 25-50 mg/kg/day (max 2 g/day) in divided doses every 6 hours for a full 10 days. **125 mg/5 mL @ 25 mg/kg/day** 10 kg (22 lb) = ½ tsp (2.5 mL) Q6H 15 kg (33 lb) = ¾ tsp Q6H 20 kg (44 lb) = 1 tsp (5 mL) Q6H	**Food:** Take 1 hour before or 2 hours after meals. May take with food if GI upset occurs. **Important side effects:** Nausea, rash.

250 mg/5 mL Q6H × 10 days <$ 500 mg PO Q8H × 10 days <$	>20 kg (44 lb) = Use adult dose. **250 mg/5 mL @ 50 mg/kg/day** 10 kg (22 lb) = ½ tsp (2.5 mL) Q6H 15 kg (33 lb) = ¾ tsp Q6H 20 kg (44 lb) = 1 tsp (5 mL) Q6H >20 kg (44 lb) = Use adult dose. **Adult:** 250 mg PO four times daily or 500 mg PO two or three times daily for 10 days.	
Penicillin G benzathine - IM may be useful if compliance is questionable. (Bicillin L-A®, Permapen®) Pregnancy: B; Lactation: Unk **Inject IM only:** 300,000 U/mL, 600,000 U/mL <$ - $	**Children <60 lb:** 600,000 U IM × 1 dose. **>60 lb:** Use adult dose. **Adult:** 1.2 mU IM × 1 dose. **Recommended if patient compliance is a concern.**	**Important side effects:** Pain at injection site. Use with caution if history of seizures.
Amoxicillin (Amoxil®) Generics available Pregnancy: B; Lactation: Safe **Caps:** 250 mg, 500 mg **Tabs:** 500 mg, 875 mg **Chew tab:** 125 mg, 200 mg, 250 mg, 400 mg **Oral Susp:** 125 mg/5 mL, 250 mg/5 mL, 400 mg/5 mL	**Children:** 45-90 mg/kg/day (max 1500 mg/day) in divided doses three times daily for 10-14 days. **250 mg/5 mL at 90 mg/kg/day** 8 kg (18 lb) = 1 tsp (5 mL) Q8H 17 kg (37 lb) = 2 tsp (10 mL) Q8H >17 kg = Use adult dose. **Adult:** 500 mg PO three times daily for 10-14 days.	**Food:** May take with or without meals. **Important side effects:** Diarrhea and nausea. May cause nonallergic maculopapular rash. **Reduce dose if renal impairment (CrCl <30 mL/min).**

(continued)

Drug, Its Forms and Dosage Increments	Children and Adult Dosages and Instructions	Information and Important Side Effects
Oral drops: 50 mg/mL <$	May be useful in children who require oral suspension due to better palatability vs. penicillin VK suspension. However, penicillin VK remains the drug of choice.	
Amoxicillin/clavulanate (Augmentin®) Pregnancy: B; Lactation: Unk **Q12H Formulations:** **Tabs:** 500 mg/125 mg, 875 mg/125 mg **Chewable Tabs:** 200 mg/28.5 mg, 400 mg/57 mg **Oral Susp:** 200 mg/28.5 mg/5 mL, 400 mg/57 mg/5 mL, 600 mg/42.9 mg/5 mL Child - $$$ Adult - >$$$$	**Children:** 45 mg amoxicillin component/kg/day (max 1600 mg/day) every 12 hours for 10-14 days. **Q12H using 200 mg/5 mL susp @ 45 mg/kg/day** 9 kg (20 lb) = 1 tsp (5 mL) Q12H 13 kg (29 lb) = 1½ tsp (7.5 mL) Q12H 18 kg (40 lb) = 2 tsp (10 mL) Q12H **Q12H using 400 mg/5 mL susp @ 45 mg/kg/day** 18 kg (40 lb) = 1 tsp (5 mL) Q12H 27 kg (59 lb) = 1½ tsp (7.5 mL) Q12H 35 kg (77 lb) = 2 tsp (10 mL) Q12H >40 kg = Use adult dose (max 875 mg Q12H). **Adult:** 500-875 mg twice daily for 10-14 days. Note: Q12H dosing may improve compliance compared to Q8H dosing.	**Food:** Take with food to reduce diarrhea. **Important side effects:** Diarrhea (common), nausea, rash. **Reduce dose if renal impairment (CrCl <30 mL/min).**
Azithromycin* (Zithromax®)	**Children ≥2 years:** 12 mg/kg/day (max 500 mg/day) once daily for 5 days.	**Food:** Oral suspension should be taken 1 hour before or 2 hours after food.

Pregnancy: B; Lactation: Unk **Tabs:** 250 mg and Z-Pak (500 mg × 1 day, then 250 mg daily × 4) **Oral Susp:** 100 mg/5 mL, 200 mg/5 mL 20-kg child - $$ Z-Pak - $$$	**100 mg/5 mL** 8-9 kg (20 lb) = 1 tsp (5 mL) Q24H **200 mg/5 mL** 18 kg (40 lb) = 1 tsp (5 mL) Q24H 25 kg (55 lb) = 1½ tsp (7.5 mL) Q24H 33 kg (73 lb) = 2 tsp (10 mL) Q24H 40 kg (88 lb) = 2½ tsp (12.5 mL) Q24H ≥40 kg (88 lb) = 500 mg Q24H **Adolescent ≥16 years and Adult:** Dispense one Z-Pak.	Tablets may be taken without regard to food. **Important side effects:** Nausea, diarrhea, elevated LFTs.
Cefpodoxime (Vantin®) Pregnancy: B; Lactation: Unk **Tabs:** 100 mg, 200 mg **Oral Susp:** 50 mg/5 mL, 100 mg/5 mL 50 mg/5 mL Q12H × 10 days - $$ 200 mg PO Q12H × 10 days - >$$$$	**Children >5 months to 12 years:** 10 mg/kg (max 200 mg/day) twice daily for 5-10 days. **50 mg/5 mL @ 10 mg/kg/day** 10 kg (22 lb) = 1 tsp (5 mL) Q12H 15 kg (33 lb) = 1½ tsp (7.5 mL) Q12H **100 mg/5 mL @10 mg/kg/day** 15 kg (33 lb) = ¾ tsp Q12H ≥20 kg (44 lb) = 1 tsp (5 mL) Q12H **Children ≥13 years to Adult:** 100-400 mg PO twice daily for 4-10 days.	**Food:** Take tablet with food. Suspension may be taken without regard to food. **Important side effects:** Diarrhea. **Reduce dose if renal impairment (CrCl <30 mL/min).**
Cefuroxime axetil (Ceftin®) Pregnancy: B; Lactation: Unsafe **Tabs:** 125 mg, 250 mg, 500 mg **Oral Susp:** 125 mg/5 mL, 250 mg/5 mL	**Children ≥3 months to 12 years:** 20 mg/kg/day (max 500 mg/day) in divided doses twice daily for 10 days. **125 mg/5 mL @ 20 mg/kg/day** 6 kg (13 lb) = ½ tsp Q12H	**Food:** Take suspension with food. Tablets may be taken without regard to food. **Important side effects:** Nausea, vomiting, diarrhea.

(continued)

Drug, Its Forms and Dosage Increments	Children and Adult Dosages and Instructions	Information and Important Side Effects
125 mg/5 mL Q12H × 10 days - $$ 250 mg PO Q12H × 10 days - >$$$$	12 kg (26 lb) = 1 tsp (5 mL) Q12H 18 kg (40 lb) = 1½ tsp Q12H 24 kg (53 lb) = 2 tsp (10 mL) Q12H **Children ≥13 years or Adult:** 250 mg PO twice daily for 10 days.	**Reduce dose if renal impairment (CrCl <30 mL/min).**
Cephalexin (Keflex®) Generics available Pregnancy: B; Lactation: Unk **Tabs:** 250 mg, 500 mg, 1 g **Caps:** 250 mg, 500 mg **Oral Susp:** 125 mg/5 mL, 250 mg/5 mL 250 mg/5 mL Q6H × 10 days - <$ 500 mg PO Q6H × 10 days - $	**Children:** 25-50 mg/kg/day (max 4 g/day) in divided doses two to four times daily for 10 days. **125 mg/5 mL @ 25 mg/kg/day** (double for 50 mg/kg) 10 kg (22 lb) = ½ tsp (2.5 mL) Q6H 15 kg (33 lb) = ¾ tsp Q6H 20 kg (44 lb) = 1 tsp (5 mL) Q6H **250 mg/5 mL @ 25 mg/kg/day** (double for 50 mg/kg) 20 kg (44 lb) = ½ tsp (2.5 mL) Q6H 40 kg (88 lb) = 1 tsp (5 mL) Q6H >40 kg = Use adult dose. **Adult:** 500 mg PO four times daily for 10 days.	**Food:** Take 1 hour before or 2 hours after meals. May take with food if GI upset occurs. **Important side effects:** GI upset, diarrhea. **Reduce dose if renal impairment (CrCl <40 mL/min).**
Clarithromycin* (Biaxin, Biaxin XL®) Pregnancy: C; Lactation: Unk **Tabs:** 250 mg, 500 mg **Extended Release Tab (XL):** 500 mg	**Children ≥6 months:** 15 mg/kg/day (max 1 g/day) in divided doses twice daily for 10-14 days. **125 mg/5 mL @15 mg/kg/day** 9 kg (20 lb) = ½ tsp (2.5 mL) Q12H	**Food:** Extended release tablet with food. Others without regard to food. **Important side effects:** Nausea, drug interactions.

Oral Susp: 125 mg/5 mL, 250 mg/5 mL 250 mg/5 mL Q12H × 10 days - $$$ 500 mg PO Q12H × 10 days - $$$$	17 kg (37 lb) = 1 tsp (5 mL) Q12H **250 mg/5 mL @ 15 mg/kg/day** 17 kg (37 lb) = ½ tsp (2.5 mL) Q12H 25 kg (55 lb) = ¾ tsp Q12H 33 kg (73 lb) = 1 tsp (5 mL) Q12H **Adult:** 500 mg PO twice daily or 1 g XL once daily for 10 days.	
Clindamycin* (Cleocin®) Generics available Pregnancy: B; Lactation: Unk **Cleocin Caps:** 75 mg, 150 mg, 300 mg **Oral Solution:** 75 mg/5 mL 150 mg/10 mL Q8H × 10 days - $$$ 300 mg PO Q6H × 10 days - $$	**Children:** 20-25 mg/kg/day (max 1.8 g/day) in divided doses three time daily for 10 days. **75 mg/5 mL @ 20 mg/kg/day divided Q8H** 6 kg (13 lb) = ½ tsp (2.5 mL) Q8H 11 kg (24 lb) = 1 tsp (5 mL) Q8H 22 kg (48 lb) = 2 tsp (10 mL) Q8H 30 kg (66 lb) = 3 tsp (15 mL) Q8H 40 kg (88 lb) = 300 mg Q8H >40 kg = Use adult dose. **Adult: Mild to moderate:** 150-300 mg PO four times daily for 10-14 days. **Severe:** 450 mg PO four times daily for 10-14 days.	**Food:** May take with or without meals. Take with full glass of water to prevent esophagitis. **Important side effects:** Diarrhea, may be severe. Nausea. **May cause severe colitis.** Encourage patient to report severe, persistent, or bloody diarrhea.
Erythromycin estolate or base* (Ilosone®, E-mycin®, Ery-Tab®) Generics available Pregnancy: B; Lactation: Unsafe	**Children:** 20-40 mg/kg/day (max 2 g/day) in two to four divided doses daily for 10-14 days. **125 mg/5 mL @ 20 mg/kg/day** 4-6 kg (10-15 lb) = ½ tsp (2.5 mL) Q12H	**Food:** May take with or without meals. Take with food if causes GI upset. **Important side effects:** GI upset, hepatitis.

(continued)

Drug, Its Forms and Dosage Increments	Children and Adult Dosages and Instructions	Information and Important Side Effects
Estolate: **Tabs:** 500 mg **Caps:** 250 mg **Oral Susp:** 125 mg/5 mL, 250 mg/5 mL **Oral Drops:** 100 mg/mL 250 mg/5 mL Q12H × 10 days - $ **Base:** **Tabs:** 250 mg, 333 mg, 500 mg **Caps:** 250 mg 500 mg PO Q6H × 10 days - $	7-11 kg (16-25 lb) = 1 tsp (5 mL) Q12H 12-16 kg (26-35 lb) = 1½ tsp (7.5 mL) Q12H **250 mg/5 mL @ 20 mg/kg/day** 17-25 kg (37-55 lb) = 1 tsp (5 mL) Q12H 26-37 kg (57-81 lb) = 1½ tsp (7.5 mL) Q12H >38 kg (83 lb) = 500 mg Q12H **Adult:** Erythromycin base or estolate 500 mg PO four times daily for 10-14 days.	

PHARYNX / NECK – Tonsillitis/Pharyngitis (*Mycoplasma pneumoniae*, *Chlamydia pneumoniae*)

Drug, Its Forms and Dosage Increments	Children and Adult Dosages and Instructions	Information and Important Side Effects
Azithromycin* (Zithromax®) Pregnancy: B; Lactation: Unk **Tabs:** 250 mg and Z-Pak (500 mg × 1 day, then 250 mg daily × 4) **Oral Susp:** 100 mg/5 mL, 200 mg/5 mL 20 kg child - $$ Z-Pak - $$$	**Children ≥6 months:** 10 mg/kg/day (max 500 mg) PO daily × 1 day, then 5 mg/kg/day (max 250 mg) PO daily × 4 days. **100 mg/5 mL** 10 kg (22 lb) = 1 tsp (5 mL) × 1 day, then ½ tsp (2.5 mL) daily for days 2-5. **200 mg/5 mL** 20 kg (44 lb) = 1 tsp (5 mL) × 1 day, then ½ tsp (2.5 mL) daily for days 2-5. 30 kg (66 lb) = 1.5 tsp × 1 day, then ¾ tsp daily for days 2-5. **Adult:** Dispense one Z-Pak.	**Food:** Oral suspension should be taken 1 hour before or 2 hours after food. Tablets may be taken without regard to food. **Important side effects:** Nausea, diarrhea, elevated LFTs.

Clarithromycin* (Biaxin, Biaxin XL®) Pregnancy: C; Lactation: Unk **Tabs:** 250 mg, 500 mg **Extend Release Tab (XL):** 500 mg **Oral Susp:** 125 mg/5 mL, 250 mg/5 mL 250 mg/5 mL Q12H × 10 days - $$$ 500 mg PO Q12H × 10 days - $$$$	**Children ≥6 months:** 15 mg/kg/day (max 1 g/day) in divided doses twice daily for 7-14 days. **125 mg/5 mL @ 15 mL/kg/day** 9 kg (20 lb) = ½ tsp (2.5 mL) Q12H 17 kg (37 lb) = 1 tsp (5 mL) Q12H **250 mg/5 mL @ 15 mL/kg/day** 17 kg (37 lb) = ½ tsp (2.5 mL) Q12H 25 kg (55 lb) = ¾ tsp Q12H 33 kg (73 lb) = 1 tsp (5 mL) Q12H **Adult:** 500 mg PO twice daily or 1 gXL PO once daily for 7-14 days.	**Food:** Extended release tablet with food. Others without regard to food. **Important side effects:** Nausea, drug interactions.
Doxycycline* (Vibramycin®) Generics available Pregnancy: D; Lactation: Unsafe **Caps:** 50 mg, 100 mg **Tabs:** 50 mg, 100 mg 10 days <$	**Adolescents ≥8 years or Adult:** 100 mg PO twice daily for 7-14 days.	**Food:** May take with food if GI upset occurs. Take 1 hour before or 2 hours after antacids, iron, milk, or other dairy products. Take with full glass of water to prevent esophagitis. **Important side effects:** Photosensitivity (use sunscreen), esophagitis. May discolor fingernails.
Erythromycin estolate or base* (Ilosone®, E-mycin®, Ery-Tab®) Generics available Pregnancy: B; Lactation: Unsafe **Estolate:** **Tabs:** 500 mg	**Children:** 20-40 mg/kg/day estolate (max 2 g/day) in two to four divided doses daily for 7-14 days. **125 mg/5 mL @ 20 mg/kg/day** 4-6 kg (10-15 lb) = ½ tsp (2.5 mL) Q12H 7-11 kg (16-25 lb) = 1 tsp (5 mL) Q12H	**Food:** May take with or without meals. Take with food if causes GI upset. **Important side effects:** GI upset, hepatitis.

(continued)

Drug, Its Forms and Dosage Increments	Children and Adult Dosages and Instructions	Information and Important Side Effects
Caps: 250 mg **Oral Susp:** 125 mg/5 mL, 250 mg/5 mL 250 mg/5 mL Q12H × 10 days - $ **Base:** **Tabs:** 250 mg, 333 mg, 500 mg **Caps:** 250 mg 500 mg PO Q6H × 10 days - $	12-16 kg (26-35 lb) = 1½ tsp (7.5 mL) Q12H **250 mg/5 mL @ 20 mg/kg/day** 17-25 kg = 1 tsp (5 mL) Q12H 26-37 kg = 1½ tsp (7.5 mL) Q12H >38 kg = 500 mg Q12H **Adult:** Erythromycin Base or Estolate 500 mg PO four times daily for 7-14 days.	

PHARYNX / NECK – Tonsillitis/Pharyngitis (*Haemophilus influenzae*)

Drug, Its Forms and Dosage Increments	Children and Adult Dosages and Instructions	Information and Important Side Effects
Azithromycin* (Zithromax®) Pregnancy: B; Lactation: Unk **Tabs:** 250 mg and Z-Pak (500 mg × 1 day, then 250 mg daily × 4) **Oral Susp:** 100 mg/5 mL, 200 mg/5 mL 20-kg child - $$ Z-Pak - $$$	**Children ≥6 months:** 10 mg/kg/day (max 500 mg) PO daily × 1 day, then 5 mg/kg/day (max 250 mg) PO daily × 4 days **100 mg/5 mL** 10 kg (22 lb) = 1 tsp (5 mL) × 1 day, then ½ tsp (2.5 mL) daily for days 2-5. **200 mg/5 mL** 20 kg (44 lb) = 1 tsp (5 mL) × 1 day, then ½ tsp (2.5 mL) daily for days 2-5. 30 kg (66 lb) = 1.5 tsp × 1 day, then ¾ tsp daily for days 2-5. **Adult:** Dispense one Z-Pak.	**Food:** Oral suspension should be taken 1 hour before or 2 hours after food. Tablets may be taken without regard to food. **Important side effects:** Nausea, diarrhea, elevated LFTs.

Drug	Dosing	Comments
Cefuroxime axetil (Ceftin®) Pregnancy: B; Lactation: Unsafe **Tabs:** 125 mg, 250 mg, 500 mg **Oral Susp:** 125 mg/5 mL, 250 mg/5 mL 125 mg/5 mL Q12H × 10 days - $$ 250 mg PO Q12H × 10 days - >$$$$	**Children >3 months to 12 years:** 30 mg/kg/day (max 1,000 mg/day) in divided doses twice daily for 10 days. **125 mg/5 mL @ 30 mg/kg/day** 8 kg (18 lb) = 1 tsp (5 mL) Q12H 12.5 kg (27 lb) = 1½ tsp (7.5 mL) Q12H 17 kg (37 lb) = 2 tsp (10 mL) Q12H 25 kg (55 lb) = 3 tsp (15 mL) Q12H 33 kg (73 lb) = Use adult dose. **Children ≥13 years or Adult:** 250-500 mg PO twice daily for 10 days.	**Food:** Take suspension with food. Tablets may be taken without regard to food. **Important side effects:** Nausea, vomiting, diarrhea. **Reduce dose in renal disease (CrCl <30 mL/min).**
Trimethoprim/Sulfamethoxazole* (Bactrim®, Septra®) Generics available Pregnancy: C; Lactation: Unsafe **Single Strength (SS) Tabs:** 80 mg/400 mg **Double Strength (DS) Tabs:** 160 mg/800 mg **Oral Susp:** 40 mg/200 mg per 5 mL 10 mL Q12H × 10 days <$ DS Tab PO Q12H × 10 days - $	**Children >2 months:** 8-10 mg/kg/day TMP component (max 320 mg/day) in divided doses twice daily for 10-14 days. **8-10 mg/kg/day @ 40 mg/200 mg/5 mL** 10 kg (22 lb) = 1 tsp (5 mL) Q12H 20 kg (44 lb) = 2 tsp (10 mL) or 1 SS Tab Q12H 30 kg (66 lb) = 3 tsp (15 mL) or 1½ SS Tab Q12H 40 kg (88 lb) = 4 tsp (20 mL) or 2 SS Tabs or 1 DS Tab Q12H **Adult:** 1 DS Tab PO twice daily for 10-14 days.	**Food:** May take without regard to food. Encourage fluids. **Important side effects:** Photosensitivity, rash. **Reduce dose in renal disease (CrCl <30 mL/min).**

(continued)

Drug, Its Forms and Dosage Increments	Children and Adult Dosages and Instructions	Information and Important Side Effects
PHARYNX / NECK – Gonococcal Pharyngitis (*Neisseria gonorrhoeae*)		
<u>Ceftriaxone</u> (IM) (Rocephin®) Pregnancy: B; Lactation: Unk **Vials:** 250 mg, 500 mg, 1,000 mg **Vials with 2.1 mL Lidocaine for IM injection:** 500 mg, 1,000 mg	**Children and Adult:** 125 mg IM × 1 dose. **Children ≥45 kg and adults treat with concomitant azithromycin or doxycycline for presumptive *C. trachomatis*.**	**Important side effects:** Pain at injection site.
Azithromycin* (Zithromax®) Pregnancy: B; Lactation: Unk **Tabs:** 250 mg - $$ **Powder for Oral Suspension:** 1 g - $$	**Children ≥45 kg and Adult:** 1 g PO × 1 dose. **Use in conjunction with ceftriaxone, ciprofloxacin, or ofloxacin.**	**Food:** Oral suspension should be taken 1 hour before or 2 hours after food. Tablets may be taken without regard to food. **Important side effects:** Nausea, diarrhea, elevated LFTs.
Ciprofloxacin* (Cipro®) Pregnancy: C; Lactation: Unsafe **Tabs:** 250 mg, 500 mg - <$	**≥18 years:** 500 mg PO × 1 dose. **Treat concomitantly with azithromycin or doxycycline for presumptive *C. trachomatis*.**	**Food:** May take with food if it causes GI upset, but avoid large amounts of dairy products. May take 2 hours before or 6 hours after sucralfate, antacids, aluminum, magnesium, calcium, zinc, iron, vitamins, or mineral supplements. **Important side effects:** Photosensitivity and dizziness.
Doxycycline* (Vibramycin®)	**Children ≥8 years and Adult:** 100 mg PO twice daily for 7 days.	**Food:** May take with food if GI upset occurs. Take 1 hour before or 2 hours

Generics available Pregnancy: D; Lactation: Unsafe **Caps:** 50 mg, 100 mg - <$ **Tabs:** 50 mg, 100 mg - <$	**Use in conjunction with ceftriaxone, ciprofloxacin, or ofloxacin.**	after antacids, iron, milk, or other dairy products. Take with full glass of water to prevent esophagitis. **Important side effects:** Photosensitivity (use sunscreen), esophagitis. May discolor fingernails.
Ofloxacin* (Floxin®) Pregnancy: C; Lactation: Unk **Tabs:** 200 mg, 300 mg, 400 mg - <$	**≥18 years:** 400 mg PO × 1 dose. **Treat concomitantly with azithromycin or doxycycline for presumptive *C. trachomatis*.**	**Food:** May take without regard to food. Do not take within 2 hours of sucralfate, antacids, aluminum, magnesium, calcium, zinc, iron, vitamins, or mineral supplements. **Important side effects:** Nausea, photosensitivity, dizziness.

PHARYNX / NECK – Gonococcal Pharyngitis in Pregnancy (*Neisseria gonorrhoeae*)

<u>Ceftriaxone</u> (IM) (Rocephin®) Pregnancy: B; Lactation: Unk	**Adolescents and Adult:** 125 mg IM × 1 dose. **Treat concomitantly with erythromycin or amoxicillin for presumptive *C. trachomatis*.**	**Important side effect:** Pain at injection site.
Amoxicillin (Amoxil®) Generics available Pregnancy: B; Lactation: Safe **Caps:** 250 mg, 500 mg - <$	**Adolescents and Adult:** 500 mg PO three times daily for 7 days. **Use in conjunction with ceftriaxone, cefixime, or spectinomycin.**	**Food:** May take with or without meals. **Important side effects:** Diarrhea and nausea. May cause nonallergic maculopapular rash.

(continued)

PHARYNX / NECK – Gonococcal Pharyngitis in Pregnancy (*Neisseria gonorrhoeae*)

Drug, Its Forms and Dosage Increments	Children and Adult Dosages and Instructions	Information and Important Side Effects
Cefixime **May be less effective than ceftriaxone in oropharyngeal infection, but is a useful oral alternative.** (Suprax®) Pregnancy: B; Lactation: Unk **Tabs:** 200 mg, 400 mg - <$	**Adolescents and Adult:** 400 mg PO × 1 dose. **Treat concomitantly with erythromycin or amoxicillin for presumptive *C. trachomatis*.**	**Food:** May be taken without regard to food. Food may reduce GI upset. **Important side effects:** Rash, nausea, diarrhea.
Erythromycin Base* (E-Mycin®, Ery-Tab®) Generics available Pregnancy: B; Lactation: Safe **Tabs:** 250 mg, 500 mg - <$ **Caps:** 250 mg - $	**Adolescents and Adult:** 500 mg PO four times daily for 7 days or if GI intolerance, 250 mg PO four times daily for 14 days. **Use in conjunction with ceftriaxone, cefixime, or spectinomycin.**	**Food:** May take with or without meals. Take with food if causes GI upset. **Important side effects:** GI upset, hepatitis.
Spectinomycin* (IM) Alternative for cephalosporin allergy. (Trobicin®) Pregnancy: B; Lactation: Unk **IM Injection:** 2 g $$	**Adolescents and Adult:** 2 g IM × 1 dose. **Treat concomitantly with erythromycin for presumptive *C. trachomatis*.**	**Important side effect:** Pain at injection site.

PHARYNX / NECK – Tonsillitis/Pharyngitis (*Corynebacterium diphtheria*)

Comment: Potentially serious disease. Requires hospital admission for antitoxin, parenteral antibiotics, and close monitoring. Penicillin and erythromycin are antibiotics of choice.

PHARYNX / NECK – Epiglottitis (*Haemophilus influenzae,* Group A *Streptococcus, Staphylococcus aureus*)

Comment: Refer immediately—medical emergency. May require emergent artificial airway management. Will require IV antibiotics.

PHARYNX / NECK – Peritonsillar Abscess (Group A *Streptococcus, Viridans streptococci, Staphylococcus aureus, anaerobes*)

Comment: Refer to ENT. Drainage required if abscess present. May need to start antibiotics if referral cannot occur urgently.

Penicillin G (Intravenous) (Pfizerpen®) Pregnancy: B; Lactation: Unk	**Children:** 100,000-400,000 U/kg/day IV in divided doses every 4 to 6 hours (max 24 mU/day). **Adolescent and Adult:** 24 mU/day IV in divided doses every 4 to 6 hours.	**Important side effects:** Diarrhea, agitation, seizures, rash, bleeding abnormalities, decreased WBC count, drug fever, superinfection. Use with caution in patients with history of seizure.
Then **Penicillin V Potassium** (Pen-Vee K® Veetids®) Generics available Pregnancy: B; Lactation: Unk **Tabs:** 250 mg, 500 mg **Powder for Oral Suspension:** 125 mg/5 mL, 250 mg/5 mL **Administer oral or IV penicillin with either oral or IV metronidazole as below.**	**Children <12 years:** 25-50 mg/kg/day in divided doses every 6 to 8 hours (max 3 g/day). **Children ≥12 years and Adult:** 500 mg PO every 6 to 8 hours.	**Food:** Take 1 hour before or 2 hours after meals. May take with food if GI upset occurs. **Important side effects:** Bad taste, GI upset, vomiting, diarrhea, agitation, seizures, rash. Use with caution in patients with history of seizures.
Metronidazole (Parenteral) (Flagyl®) Generics available Pregnancy: B; Lactation: Unsafe	**Children:** 30 mg/kg/day IV in divided doses every 6 hours (max 4 g/day). **Adult:** 1,000 mg IV load, then 500 mg IV every 6 hours.	

(continued)

Drug, Its Forms and Dosage Increments	Children and Adult Dosages and Instructions	Information and Important Side Effects
Then **Metronidazole** (Flagyl®) Generics available Pregnancy: B; Lactation: Unsafe **Tabs:** 250 mg, 500 mg - <$ ***Administer metronidazole with penicillin as above.**	**Children:** 30 mg/kg/day PO in divided doses every 6 hours (max 4 g/day). **Adult:** 30 mg/kg/day (max 4 g/day), usually 500-1,000 mg PO every 6 hours.	**Food:** Administer on empty stomach unless GI upset occurs, then with food. **Important side effects:** Dizziness, headache, confusion, seizures, nausea, metallic taste, insomnia, paresthesias. May cause disulfiram—like reaction-avoid alcohol. Use cautiously in persons with history of seizure disorder.
Clindamycin* (Cleocin®) Generics available Pregnancy: B; Lactation: Unk **Caps:** 75 mg, 150 mg, - $$ 300 mg - >$$$$ **Oral Solution:** 75 mg/5 mL - $	**Children: Mild to Moderate:** 10-15 mg/kg/day (max 1.8 g/day) PO in divided doses three or four times daily for 14 days. **Severe:** 16-30 mg/kg/day (max 1.8 g/day) in divided doses three or four times daily for 14 days. **75 mg/5 mL @ 10 mg/kg/day divided Q8H.** 10 kg (22 lb) = ½ tsp (2.5 mL) Q8H 20 kg (44 lb) = 1 tsp (5 mL) Q8H 30 kg (66 lb) = 1½ tsp (7.5 mL) Q8H 40 kg (88 lb) = 2 tsp (10 mL) Q8H >40 kg = Use adult dose. **Adult: Mild to Moderate:** 150-300 mg PO three to four times daily for 10-14 days. **Severe:** 450 mg PO four times daily for 10-14 days.	**Food:** May take with or without meals. Take with full glass of water to prevent esophagitis. **Important side effects:** Diarrhea, may be severe. Nausea. **May cause severe colitis.** Encourage patient to report severe, persistent, or bloody diarrhea.

MOUTH – Dental Infections (*Viridans streptococci*, Group A *Streptococcus*, anaerobes)

Drug	Dosing	Comments
Penicillin V Potassium (Pen-Vee K®) Generics available Pregnancy: B; Lactation: Unsafe **Tabs:** 125 mg, 250 mg, 500 mg **Oral Susp:** 125 mg/5 mL, 250 mg/5 mL 250 mg/5 mL Q6H × 10 days <$ 500 mg PO Q8H × 10 days <$ **Strongly consider adding metronidazole for moderate to severe infection.**	**Children <12 years:** 25-50 mg/kg/day (max 2 g/day) in divided doses every 6 hours for 10-14 days. **125 mg/5 mL @ 25 mg/kg/day** 10 kg (22 lb) = ½ tsp (2.5 mL) Q6H 15 kg (33 lb) = ¾ tsp Q6H 20 kg (44 lb) = 1 tsp (5 mL) Q6H >20 kg (44 lb) = Use adult dose. **250 mg/5 mL @ 50 mg/kg/day** 10 kg (22 lb) = ½ tsp (2.5 mL) Q6H 15 kg (33 lb) = ¾ tsp Q6H 20 kg (44 lb) = 1 tsp (5 mL) Q6H >20 kg (44 lb) = Use adult dose. **Children ≥12 years to Adult:** 250 mg PO four times daily or 500 mg PO two to three times daily for 10-14 days.	**Food:** Take 1 hour before or 2 hours after meals. May take with food if GI upset occurs. **Important side effects:** Nausea, rash. Use with caution if history of seizures.
Metronidazole* (Flagyl®) Generics available Pregnancy: B; Lactation: Unk **Tabs:** 250 mg, 500 mg - <$ **Use in conjunction with penicillin.**	**Children:** 30 mg/kg/day in divided doses 3 or 4 times daily (max 4 g/day) 10 kg (22 lb) = ½ tsp (2.5 mL) Q6H 15 kg (33 lb) = ¾ tsp Q6H 20 kg (44 lb) = 1 tsp (5 mL) Q6H **Adult:** 250-500 mg PO every 6 hours.	**Food:** Administer on empty stomach unless GI upset occurs, then with food. **Important side effects:** Dizziness, headache, confusion, seizures, nausea, metallic taste, insomnia, paresthesias. Avoid alcohol. Use with caution in persons with history of seizure disorder.

(continued)

MOUTH – Dental Infections (*Viridans streptococci*, Group A *Streptococcus*, anaerobes)

Drug, Its Forms and Dosage Increments	Children and Adult Dosages and Instructions	Information and Important Side Effects
Clindamycin* (Cleocin®) Generics available Pregnancy: B; Lactation: Unk **Caps:** 75 mg, 150 mg, 300 mg **Oral Solution:** 75 mg/5 mL 150 mg/10 mL Q8H × 10 days - $$$ 300 mg PO Q6H × 10 days - $$	**Children mild to moderate:** 10-15 mg/kg/day (max 1.8 g/day) PO in divided doses 3 or 4 times daily for 10-14 days. **Severe:** 16-30 mg/kg/day (max 1.8 g/day) in divided doses 3 or 4 times daily for 10-14 days. **75 mg/5 mL @ 10 mg/kg/day divided Q8H.** 10 kg (22 lb) = ½ tsp (2.5 mL) Q8H 20 kg (44 lb) = 1 tsp (5 mL) Q8H 30 kg (66 lb) = 1½ tsp (7.5 mL) Q8H 40 kg (88 lb) = 2 tsp (10 mL) Q8H >40 kg = Use adult dose. **Adult mild to moderate:** 150-300 mg PO 3 or 4 times daily for 10-14 days. **Severe:** 450 mg PO 4 times daily for 10-14 days.	**Food:** May take with or without meals. Take with full glass of water to prevent esophagitis. **Important side effects:** Diarrhea—may be severe. Nausea. **May cause severe colitis.** Encourage patient to report severe, persistent, or bloody diarrhea.

MOUTH – Dental Procedure Prophylaxis for Endocarditis (*Viridans streptococci*)

Drug, Its Forms and Dosage Increments	Children and Adult Dosages and Instructions	Information and Important Side Effects
Amoxicillin (Amoxil®) Pregnancy: B; Lactation: Unk **Caps:** 250 mg, 500 mg **Tabs:** 500 mg, 875 mg **Chewable Tabs:** 125 mg, 250 mg **Susp:** 125 mg/5 mL, 250 mg/5 mL	**Children:** 50 mg/kg 1 hour before procedure. **Adult:** 2 g PO 1 hour before procedure.	**Food:** May take with or without meals. **Important side effects:** Diarrhea and nausea. May cause nonallergic maculopapular rash.

MOUTH – Dental Procedure Prophylaxis for Endocarditis – Penicillin Allergic Patients
(Viridans streptococci)

Drug	Dosage	Notes
Azithromycin* (Zithromax®) Pregnancy: B; Lactation: Unk **Tabs:** 250 mg and Z-Pak (500 mg × 1 day, then 250 mg daily × 4) **Oral Susp:** 100 mg/5 mL, 200 mg/5 mL	**Children:** 15 mg/kg PO 1 hour before procedure. **Adult:** 500 mg PO 1 hour before procedure.	**Food:** Oral suspension should be taken 1 hour before or 2 hours after food. Tablets may be taken without regard to food. **Important side effects:** Nausea, diarrhea.
Cefadroxil (Duricef) Pregnancy: B; Lactation: Unk **Caps:** 500 mg, 1 g **Susp:** 125 mg/5 mL, 250 mg/5 mL, 500 mg/5 mL	**Children:** 50 mg/kg PO 1 hour before procedure. **Adult:** 2 g PO 1 hour before procedure.	**Food:** May be taken without regard to food. May take with food to reduce GI upset. **Important side effects:** Nausea, vomiting, rash, diarrhea. **Caution:** Do not use in true hypersensitivity penicillin reactions.
Cephalexin (Keflex®) Generics available Pregnancy: B; Lactation: Unk **Tabs:** 250 mg, 500 mg, 1 g **Caps:** 250 mg, 500 mg **Susp:** 125 mg/5 mL, 250 mg/5 mL	**Children:** 50 mg/kg PO 1 hour before procedure. **Adult:** 2 g PO 1 hour before procedure.	**Food:** Take 1 hour before or 2 hours after meals. May take with food if GI upset occurs. **Important side effects:** GI upset, diarrhea. **Caution:** Do not use in true hypersensitivity penicillin reactions.
Clarithromycin* (Biaxin®) Pregnancy: C; Lactation: Unk	**Children:** 15 mg/kg PO 1 hour before procedure. **Adult:** 500 mg PO 1 hour before procedure.	**Food:** Without regard to food. **Important side effects:** Nausea.

(continued)

Drug, Its Forms and Dosage Increments	Children and Adult Dosages and Instructions	Information and Important Side Effects
Tabs: 250 mg, 500 mg **Oral Susp:** 125 mg/5 mL, 250 mg/5 mL		
Clindamycin* (Cleocin®) Generics available Pregnancy: B; Lactation: Unk **Cleocin Caps:** 75 mg, 150 mg, 300 mg **Peds Oral Susp:** 75 mg/5 mL	**Children:** 20 mg/kg (max 600 mg) PO 1 hour before procedure. **Adult:** 600 mg PO 1 hour before procedure.	**Food:** May take with or without meals. Take with full glass of water to prevent esophagitis. **Important side effects:** Diarrhea (may be severe), nausea.

MOUTH – Dental Procedure Prophylaxis for Endocarditis – Patients Unable to Take Oral Medications (*Viridans streptococci*)

Drug, Its Forms and Dosage Increments	Children and Adult Dosages and Instructions	Information and Important Side Effects
Ampicillin (Principen®, Omnipen®) Generics available Pregnancy: B; Lactation: Unk	**Children:** 50 mg/kg (max 2 g) IV or IM 30 minutes before procedure. **Adult:** 2 g IV or IM 30 minutes before procedure.	**Important side effects:** Diarrhea, nausea, seizures, rash.

MOUTH – Dental Procedure Prophylaxis for Endocarditis – Penicillin Allergic and Unable to Take Oral Medications (*Viridans streptococci*)

Drug, Its Forms and Dosage Increments	Children and Adult Dosages and Instructions	Information and Important Side Effects
Cefazolin (Ancef®, Kefzol®) Pregnancy: B; Lactation: Unk	**Children:** 25 mg/kg (max 1 g) IV or IM 30 minutes before procedure. **Adult:** 1 g IV or IM 30 minutes before procedure.	**Important side effects: IM**—Pain at injection site, induration. **IV**—Phlebitis, thrombophlebitis. **Caution:** Do not use if history of true penicillin hypersensitivity reactions.

Clindamycin* (Cleocin®) Generics available Pregnancy: B; Lactation: Unk	**Children:** 20 mg/kg (max 600 mg) IV 30 minutes before procedure. **Adult:** 600 mg IV 30 minutes before procedure.	**Caution:** Do not administer >30 mg/min.

MOUTH – Esophagitis, Candidal (*Candida albicans*)

Ketoconazole* (Nizoral®) Generics available Pregnancy: C; Lactation: Unsafe **Tabs:** 200 mg - <$	**Adult:** 200-400 mg Q24H × 14-21 days.	**Food:** May take without regard to food. May take with food if GI upset occurs. Avoid taking within 2 hours of acid-suppressing drugs. **Important side effects:** Headache, dizziness, nausea, vomiting, hepatotoxicity, rash, urticaria, pruritus, reduced testosterone levels, gynecomastia.
Fluconazole* (Diflucan®) Pregnancy: C; Lactation: Unsafe **Tabs:** 50 mg, 100 mg, 150 mg, 200 mg **Oral Susp:** 10 mg/mL, 40 mg/mL in 35-mL bottles	**Adult:** 200 mg × 1, then 100 mg Q24H × 10-21 days	**Food:** May be taken without regard to food. **Side effects:** Nausea, dizziness, hepatitis, rash (potentially exfoliative). Encourage patient to report rash or nausea, epigastric discomfort, yellowing of eye(s) or skin, or easy bruising.

MOUTH – Herpes, Oral (Herpes simplex virus type 1)

Acyclovir (Zovirax®) Generics available	**Children:** (>2 years and <40 kg) 20 mg/kg/day (max of 800 mg/day) in divided doses 4 times daily for 5 days.	**Food:** May take without regard to food. Maintain good hydration.

(continued)

Drug, Its Forms and Dosage Increments	Children and Adult Dosages and Instructions	Information and Important Side Effects
Pregnancy: C; Lactation: Safe **Caps:** 200 mg - <$ **Tabs:** 400 mg, 800 mg **Suspension:** 200 mg/5 mL	(>2 years and >40 kg) 200 mg 4 times daily for 5 days. **200 mg/ 5 mL @ 20 mg/kg/day** 10 kg (22 lb) = 1.2 mL Q6H 15 kg (33 lb) = 1.8 mL Q6H 20 kg (44 lb) = 2.5 mL Q6H **Adults:** 200 mg 4 to 5 times daily for 5-10 days.	**Important side effects:** Headache, dizziness, nausea, seizures, bone-marrow suppression, nephrotoxicity. **Reduce dose in severe renal disease (CrCl <10 mL/min).**
Famciclovir* (Famvir®) Pregnancy: B; Lactation: Unsafe **Tabs:** 125 mg, 250 mg, 500 mg >$$$$	**Adult:** 500 mg PO 3 times daily for 5 days.	**Food:** May be taken without regard to food. **Important side effects:** Nausea, diarrhea, headache, dizziness, insomnia, fatigue, rash. **Reduce dose in renal disease (CrCl <60 mL/min).**
Valacyclovir (Valtrex®) Pregnancy: B; Lactation: Unk **Tabs:** 500 mg, 1,000 mg - $$$	**Adult:** First episode 1,000 mg PO twice daily for 5-7 days. **Recurrent:** 500 mg PO twice daily for 5-7 days.	**Food:** May be taken without regard to food. Maintain good hydration. **Important side effects:** Nausea, headache, diarrhea, dizziness, renal dysfunction, Hemolytic-Uremic Syndromes/Thrombocytopenia Purpura. **Reduce dose in renal disease (CrCl <30 mL/min).**

MOUTH – Oral Herpes, Pregnancy (Herpes simplex virus type 1) Use of acyclovir and valacyclovir in pregnancy are under investigation but preliminary evidence has not found them to be detrimental to the fetus. Pregnant women who receive these drugs should be reported to the CDC/Glaxo Wellcome registry (800) 722-9292, extension 38465.

Acyclovir* (Zovirax®) Pregnancy: C; Lactation: Safe **Caps:** 200 mg - **Tabs:** 400, 800 mg	**Adult:** 200 mg 4 to 5 times daily for 5-10 days.	**Food:** May take without regard to food. **Important side effects:** Headache, dizziness, nausea, seizures, bone-marrow suppression, nephrotoxicity. **Reduce dose in severe renal disease (CrCl <10 mL/min).**
Valacyclovir* (Valtrex®) Pregnancy: B; Lactation: Unk **Tabs:** 500 mg, 1,000 mg - $$$$	**Adult:** First episode 1,000 mg PO twice daily for 5-7 days. **Recurrent:** 500 mg PO twice daily for 5-7 days.	**Food:** May be taken without regard to food. Maintain good hydration. **Important side effects:** Nausea, headache, diarrhea, dizziness, renal dysfunction, HUS/TTP. **Reduce dose in severe renal disease (CrCl <30 mL/min).**
Acyclovir Topical 5% Pregnancy: C; Lactation Unk **Topical 5%**	**Adult:** Apply to lesions on lips 6 times daily for 7 days.	

MOUTH – Parotitis (*Staphylococcus aureus*) **Comment:** Oral drug therapy may be appropriate for early or mild cases. More advanced cases may require surgical drainage ± parenteral antibiotics.

Dicloxacillin (Dynapen®) Generics available	**Children ≤40 kg:** 25-50 mg/kg/day (max 2 g/day) PO in divided doses every 6 hours for 10-14 days.	**Food:** Take 1 hour before or 2 hours after meals.

(continued)

Drug, Its Forms and Dosage Increments	Children and Adult Dosages and Instructions	Information and Important Side Effects
Pregnancy: B; Lactation: Unk **Caps:** 125 mg, 250 mg, 500 mg **Oral Susp:** 62.5 mg/5 mL, 200 mL - $ Adult 10-14 days - $	**62.5 mg/5 mL @ 25 mg/kg/day** (double for 50 mg) 10 kg (22 lb) = 1 tsp (5 mL) Q6H 15 kg (33 lb) = 1½ tsp (7.5 mL) Q6H 20 kg (44 lb) = 2 tsp (10 mL) Q6H 40 kg (88 lb) = Use adult dose. **Children ≥40 kg and Adult:** 500 mg PO four times daily for 10-14 days.	**Important side effects:** Bad taste, GI upset, vomiting, diarrhea.
Clindamycin* (Cleocin®) Generics available Pregnancy: B; Lactation: Unk **Caps:** 75 mg, 150 mg, 300 mg **Oral Solution:** 75 mg/5 mL 150 mg/10 mL Q8H × 10 days - $$$ 300 mg PO Q6H × 10 days - $$	**Children: Mild to Moderate:** 10-15 mg/kg/day (max 1.8 g/day) PO in divided doses three or four times daily for 10-14 days. **Severe:** 16-30 mg/kg/day (max 1.8 g/day) in divided doses three or four times daily for 10-14 days. **75 mg/5 mL @ 10 mg/kg/day divided Q8H** 10 kg (22 lb) = ½ tsp (2.5 mL) Q8H 20 kg (44 lb) = 1 tsp (5 mL) Q8H 30 kg (66 lb) = 1½ tsp (7.5 mL) Q8H 40 kg (88 lb) = 2 tsp (10 mL) Q8H >40 kg = Use adult dose. **Adult: Mild to moderate:** 150-300 mg PO three to four times daily for 10-14 days. **Severe:** 450 mg PO four times daily for 10-14 days.	**Food:** May take with or without meals. Take with full glass of water to prevent esophagitis. **Important side effects:** Diarrhea, may be severe. Nausea. **May cause severe colitis.** Encourage patient to report severe, bloody, or persistent diarrhea.

MOUTH – Thrush (*Candida albicans*)

Drug	Dosing	Comments
Nystatin* (Mycostatin®, Nilstat®) Generics available Pregnancy: B; Lactation: Safe **Oral Susp:** 100,000 U/mL - <$ **Oral Pastilles (lozenge):** 200,000	**Newborns:** 100,000 U/mL – ½ mL in each cheek four times daily for 10-14 days. **Infants:** 100,000 U/mL – 1 mL in each cheek four times daily for 10-14 days. **Children:** 100,000 U/mL – 3 mL in each cheek four times daily **OR** 1-2 pastilles four to five times a day for 10-14 days. **Adult:** 4-6 mL swish/swallow four times daily **OR** 1-2 pastilles four to five times a day for 10-14 days. **Retain in mouth as long as possible. Pastilles should be dissolved slowly.**	**Side effects:** Diarrhea.
Clotrimazole* (Mycelex®) Pregnancy: C; Lactation: Unk **Troche:** 10 mg - <$	**Children ≥3 years and Adults:** Dissolve one troche in mouth slowly (15-30 minutes) five times daily for 7-10 days or until 2-3 days after symptoms clear.	**Side effects:** Nausea, unpleasant sensation in mouth, elevated LFTs.
Fluconazole* (Diflucan®) Pregnancy: C; Lactation: Unsafe **Tabs:** 50 mg, 100 mg, 150 mg, 200 mg - <$$$$ **Oral Susp:** 10 mg/mL in 35-mL Bottle - $$ 40 mg/mL in 35-mL bottles - >$$$$	**Children:** 6 mg/kg (max 200 mg) PO once × 1 day, then 3 mg/kg/day (max 100 mg) PO daily for 13 days. **10 mg/mL @ 3 mg/kg/day** (double for 6 mg/kg) 10 kg (22 lb) = 3 mL Q24H 15 kg (33 lb) = 4½ mL Q24H 20 kg (44 lb) = 6 mL Q24H	**Food:** May be taken without regard to food. **Side effects:** Nausea, dizziness, hepatitis rash (potentially exfoliative). Encourage patient to report rash or nausea, epigastric discomfort, yellowing of eye(s) or skin, or easy bruising.

(continued)

Drug, Its Forms and Dosage Increments	Children and Adult Dosages and Instructions	Information and Important Side Effects
	40 mg/mL @ 3 mg/kg/day (double for 6 mg/kg) 20 kg (44 lb) = 1½ mL Q24H 30 kg (66 lb) = 2.5 mL (½ tsp) Q24H or 100 mg tablet **Adult:** 200 mg PO once, then 100 mg daily for 10-14 days.	

BRONCHOPULMONARY – Bronchitis, Acute (*Streptococcus pneumoniae, Haemophilus influenzae, Moraxella catarrhalis*)

Comment: Most cases of acute bronchitis are caused by viral infection and do not require antibiotic therapy.

Drug, Its Forms and Dosage Increments	Children and Adult Dosages and Instructions	Information and Important Side Effects
Amoxicillin/clavulanate (Augmentin®) Pregnancy: B; Lactation: Unk **Q12H Formulations:** **Tabs:** 500 mg/125 mg, 875 mg/125 mg **Chewable Tabs:** 200 mg/28.5 mg, 400 mg/57 mg **Oral Susp:** 200 mg/28.5 mg/5 mL Child - $$$ Adult - >$$$$	**Children:** 45 mg amoxicillin component/kg/day (max 1600 mg/day) every 12 hours for 5-7 days. **Q12H using 200 mg/5 mL susp @ 45 mg/kg/day** 9 kg (20 lb) = 1 tsp (5 mL) Q12H 13 kg (29 lb) = 1½ tsp (7.5 mL) Q12H 18 kg (40 lb) = 2 tsp (10 mL) Q12H **Q12H using 400 mg/5 mL susp @ 45 mg/kg/day** 18 kg (40 lb) = 1 tsp (5 mL) Q12H 27 kg (59 lb) = 1½ tsp (7.5 mL) Q12H 35 kg (77 lb) = 2 tsp (10 mL) Q12H >40 kg = Use adult dose (max 875 mg Q12H)	**Food:** Take with food to reduce diarrhea. **Important side effects:** Diarrhea (common), nausea, rash. **Use with caution in hepatic disease.** **Reduce dose in renal disease (CrCl <30 mL/min).**

	Adult: 500-875 mg twice daily for 5-7 days. Note: Q12H dosing may improve compliance compared to Q8H dosing.	
Azithromycin* (Zithromax®) Pregnancy: B; Lactation: Unk **Tabs:** 250 mg and Z-Pak (500 mg × 1 day, then 250 mg daily × 4) **Oral Susp:** 100 mg/5 mL, 200 mg/5 mL 20-kg child - $$ Z-Pak - $$$	**Children ≥2 years:** 12 mg/kg/day (max 500 mg) daily for 5 days. **100 mg/5 mL** 10 kg (22 lb) = 1¼ tsp Q24H **200 mg/5 mL** 20 kg (44 lb) = 1¼ tsp Q24H 30 kg (66 lb) = 1¾ tsp Q24H ≥40 kg (88 lb) = 500 mg Q24H **Adolescent ≥16 years and Adult:** Dispense one Z-Pak.	**Food:** Oral suspension should be taken 1 hour before or 2 hours after food. Tablets may be taken without regard to food. **Important side effects:** Nausea, diarrhea, elevated LFTs.
Clarithromycin* (Biaxin, Biaxin XL®) Pregnancy: C; Lactation: Unk **Tabs:** 250 mg, 500 mg **Extended Release Tab (XL):** 500 mg **Oral Susp:** 125 mg/5 mL, 250 mg/5 mL 250 mg/5 mL Q12H × 10 days - $$$ 500 mg PO Q12H × 10 days - $$$$	**Children ≥6 months:** 15 mg/kg/day (max 1 g/day) in divided doses twice daily for 7-10 days. **125 mg/5 mL** 9 kg (20 lb) = ½ tsp (2.5 mL) Q12H 17 kg (37 lb) = 1 tsp (5 mL) Q12H **250 mg/5 mL** 25 kg (55 lb) = ¾ tsp Q12H 33 kg (73 lb) = 1 tsp (5 mL) Q12H **Adult:** 500 mg PO twice daily or 1 g XL PO once daily for 7-10 days.	**Food:** Extended release tablet with food. Others without regard to food. **Important side effects:** Nausea, drug interactions.

(continued)

Drug, Its Forms and Dosage Increments	Children and Adult Dosages and Instructions	Information and Important Side Effects
Erythromycin estolate or base* (Ilosone®, E-mycin®, Ery-Tab®) Generics available Pregnancy: B; Lactation: Unsafe **Estolate:** **Tabs:** 500 mg **Caps:** 250 mg **Susp:** 125 mg/5 mL and 250 mg/5 mL, 250 mg/5 mL Q12H × 10 days - $ **Base:** **Tabs:** 250 mg, 333 mg, 500 mg **Caps:** 250 mg 500 mg PO Q6H × 10 days - $	**Children:** 20-40 mg/kg/day estolate (max 2 g/day) PO in two to four divided doses daily for 7-10 days. **125 mg/5 mL @ 20-40 mg/kg/day** 4-6 kg (10-15 lb) = ½ tsp (2.5 mL) Q12H 7-11 kg (16-25 lb) = 1 tsp (5 mL) Q12H 12-16 kg (26-35 lb) = 1½ tsp (7.5 mL) Q12H or 1 tsp (5 mL) Q8H **250 mg/5 mL @ 20-40 mg/kg/day** 17-25 kg (37-55 lb) = 1 tsp (5 mL) Q12H 26-37 kg (57-81 lb) = 1½ tsp (7.5 mL) Q12H or 1 tsp (5 mL) Q8H ≥38 kg (84 lb) = 500 mg Q12H **Adult:** Erythromycin base or estolate 250-500 mg PO four times daily for 7-10 days.	**Food:** May take with or without meals. Take with food if causes GI upset. **Important side effects:** GI upset, hepatitis.
Trimethoprim/Sulfamethoxazole* (Bactrim®, Septra®) Generics available Pregnancy: C; Lactation: Unsafe **Single Strength (SS)Tabs:** 80 mg/400 mg **Double Strength (DS) Tabs:** 160 mg/800 mg **Oral Susp:** 40 mg/200 mg per 5 mL	**Children >2 months:** 8-12 mg/kg/day TMP component (max 320 mg/day) in divided doses twice daily for 7-10 days. **8 mg/kg/day @ 40 mg/200 mg/5 mL** 10 kg (22 lb) = 1 tsp (5 mL) Q12H 20 kg (44 lb) = 2 tsp (10 mL) or 1 SS Tab Q12H 30 kg (66 lb) = 3 tsp (15 mL) or 1½ SS Tab Q12H	**Food:** May take without regard to food. Encourage fluids. **Important side effects:** Photosensitivity, rash. **Reduce dose in severe renal disease (CrCl <30 mL/min).**

10 mL Q12H × 10 days <$ DS Tab PO Q12H × 10 days - $	40 kg (88 lb) = 4 tsp (20 mL) or 2 SS Tabs or 1 DS Tab Q12H for 10 days. **Adult:** 1 DS tablet PO twice daily for 7-10 days.	

Bronchopulmonary – Acute Bacterial Exacerbation of Chronic Bronchitis, Without Comorbid Illnesses (*Haemophilus influenzae, Moraxella catarrhalis, Streptococcus pneumoniae*) (Value of antibiotic therapy in immunocompetent patients is debatable and generally discouraged.)

Amoxicillin (Amoxil®) Generics available Pregnancy: B; Lactation: Safe **Caps:** 250, 500 mg **Tabs:** 500 mg, 875 mg $	**Adult:** 500 mg PO three times daily or 875 mg two times daily for 10 days.	**Food:** May take with or without meals. **Important side effects:** Diarrhea and nausea. May cause nonallergic maculopapular rash. **Reduce dose in severe renal disease (CrCl <30 mL/min).**
Ampicillin Principen®, Omnipen® Generics available Pregnancy: B; Lactation: Unknown **Caps:** 250 mg - <$ 500 mg - <$	**Adults:** 500 mg PO four times daily × 10 days.	**Food:** Administer on an empty stomach 1-2 hours before food. **Important side effects:** Nausea, vomiting, diarrhea, agitation, seizures, rash, bleeding abnormalities, decreased WBC count, drug fever, superinfection. **Reduce dose in severe renal disease (CrCl <30 mL/min).**
Azithromycin* (Zithromax®) Pregnancy: B; Lactation: Unk	**Adult:** Dispense one Z-Pak.	**Food:** Tablets may be taken without regard to food. **Important side effects:** Nausea, diarrhea, elevated LFTs.

(continued)

Drug, Its Forms and Dosage Increments	Children and Adult Dosages and Instructions	Information and Important Side Effects
Tabs: 250 mg and Z-Pak (500 mg × 1 day, then 250 mg daily × 4) Z-Pak - $$$		
Cefpodoxime (Vantin®) Pregnancy: B; Lactation: Unk **Tabs:** 100 mg - $$$$ 200 mg - >$$$$	**Adult:** 200 mg PO two times daily for 10 days.	**Food:** Take tablet with food. Suspension may be taken without regard to food. **Important side effects:** Nausea, vomiting, rash, diarrhea, elevated LFTs.
Clarithromycin* (Biaxin, Biaxin XL®) Pregnancy: C; Lactation: Unk **Tabs:** 250 mg, 500 mg **Extended Release Tab (XL):** 500 mg 500 mg Q12H × 10 days - $$$$	**Adult:** 500 mg twice daily or 1 g XL once daily for 10 days.	**Food:** Extended release tablet with food. Others without regard to food. **Important side effects:** Nausea, drug interactions. **Reduce dose in severe renal disease (CrCl <30 mL/min).**
Doxycycline* (Vibramycin®) Generics available Pregnancy: D; Lactation: Unsafe **Caps:** 50 mg, 100 mg **Tabs:** 50 mg, 100 mg <$	**Adult:** 100 mg PO twice daily for 10 days. May not be active against *H. influenzae.*	**Food:** May take with food if GI upset occurs. Take 1 hour before or 2 hours after antacids, iron, milk, or other dairy products. Take with full glass of water to prevent esophagitis. **Important side effects:** Photosensitivity, (use sunscreen), esophagitis. May discolor fingernails.
Trimethoprim/Sulfamethoxazole* (Bactrim®, Septra®) Generics available	**Adult:** 1 DS tablet PO twice daily for 10 days.	**Food:** May take without regard to food. **Important side effects:** Photosensitivity, rash.

Pregnancy: C; Lactation: Unsafe **Single Strength (SS)Tabs:** 80 mg/400 mg **Double Strength (DS) Tabs:** 160 mg/800 mg <$		**Reduce dose in severe renal disease (CrCl <30 mL/min).**

BRONCHOPULMONARY – Acute Bacterial Exacerbation of Chronic Bronchitis, With Comorbid Illnesses (i.e., CHF, diabetes, CRF, chronic liver disease, >65 years, four exacerbations a year) (*Haemophilus influenzae, Moraxella catarrhalis, Streptococcus pneumoniae*) **Comment:** Typically affects smokers or ex-smokers. This group often has risk factors for treatment failure and resistant bacteria. Often responds to oral prednisone. (Value of antibiotic therapy in immunocompetent patients is debatable.)

Amoxicillin/clavulanate (Augmentin®) Pregnancy: B; Lactation: Unk **Q12H Formulations:** **Tabs:** 500 mg/125 mg, 875 mg/125 mg Child - $$$ Adult - >$$$$	**Adult:** 500-875 mg twice daily for 10 days.	**Food:** Take with food to reduce diarrhea. **Important side effects:** Diarrhea (common), nausea, rash. **Reduce dose in severe renal disease (CrCl <30 mL/min).**
Ciprofloxacin* **If suspect *Pseudomonas*** (Cipro®) Pregnancy: C; Lactation: Unsafe **Tabs:** 250 mg - $$$$ 500 mg - >$$$$ 750 mg - >$$$$	**≥18 years to Adult:** 500-750 mg twice daily for 10 days.	**Food:** May take with food if it causes GI upset, but avoid large amounts of dairy products. May take 2 hours before or 6 hours after sucralfate, antacids, aluminum, magnesium, calcium, zinc, iron, vitamins, or mineral supplements. **Important side effects:** Photosensitivity, dizziness, headache, insomnia. *(continued)*

Drug, Its Forms and Dosage Increments	Children and Adult Dosages and Instructions	Information and Important Side Effects
		Reduce dose in severe renal disease (CrCl <50 mL/min).
Gatifloxacin* Tequin® Pregnancy: C; Lactation: Unsafe **Tabs:** 200 mg - >$$$$ 400 mg - >$$$$	**≥18 years to Adult:** 400 mg PO once daily for 7-10 days.	**Food:** May take without regard to food. Do not take within 4 hours of sucralfate, antacids, vitamins, or mineral products. **Important side effects:** Photosensitivity, dizziness, headache. **Reduce dose in severe renal disease (CrCl <40 mL/min).**
Levofloxacin* (Levaquin®) Pregnancy: C; Lactation: Unsafe **Tabs:** 250 mg, 500 mg - >$$$$	**Adult:** 500 mg PO once daily for 7-10 days.	**Food:** May take without regard to food. Do not take within 2 hours of sucralfate, antacids, aluminum, magnesium, calcium, zinc, iron, vitamins, or mineral supplements. **Important side effects:** Photosensitivity, dizziness. **Reduce dose in severe renal disease (CrCl <50 mL/min).**
Moxifloxacin* (Avelox®) Pregnancy: C; Lactation: Unsafe **Tabs:** 400 mg - >$$$$	**≥18 years to Adult:** 400 mg PO once daily 5 days.	**Food:** May take without regard to food. Must take 4 hours before or 8 hours after sucralfate, antacids, aluminum, magnesium, calcium, zinc, iron, vitamins, or mineral supplements.

		Important side effects: Photosensitivity, dizziness, headache, insomnia.

BRONCHOPULMONARY – Influenza (*Haemophilus influenzae* types A, B)

Amantadine* (Influenza A only) (Symmetrel®) Pregnancy: C; Lactation: Unk **Caps:** 100 mg **Tabs:** 100 mg **Syrup:** 50 mg/5 mL 5 days - >$	**Children (1-9 years):** 5 mg/kg/day twice daily (max 150 mg/day) × 5 days **Children (10-12 years):** 5 mg/kg/day twice daily (max 200 mg/day) × 5 days 50 mg/mL @ 5 mg/kg/day 5 kg (11 lb) = ¼ tsp Q12H 10 kg (22 lb) = ½ tsp (2.5 mL) Q12H 15 kg (33 lb) = ¾ tsp Q12H 20 kg (44 lb) = 1 tsp (5 mL) Q12H **Adult:** 13-64 years: 100 mg Q12H × 5 days **Adult >65:** 100 mg once daily × 5 days	**Food:** With or without meals. Avoid excessive alcohol. **Important side effects:** Anxiety, nervousness, nausea.
Oseltamivir (Influenza A and B) (Tamiflu®) Pregnancy: C; Lactation: Unk **Caps:** 75 mg **Powder:** 12 mg/mL (100 mL) 5 days - $$$	**Children 1-12 years:** × 5 days. **12 mg/mL Suspension** <15 kg (33 lb) = 2.5 mL Q12H <15-23 kg (34-50 lb) = 3.8 mL Q12H >23-40 kg (50-88 lb) = 5 mL Q12H >40 kg (88 lb) = 6.2 mL Q12H **Adult:** 75 mg Q12H × 5 days.	**Food:** With or without meals. **Important side effects:** Nausea, vomiting that can be reduced with food.
Rimantadine (Influenza A only) (Flumadine®) Pregnancy: C; Lactation: Unk **Tabs:** 100 mg	**Children:** Rimantadine is only approved for prophylaxis in young children. However, experts consider it appropriate for treatment of influenza in children of all ages.	**Food:** With or without meals. **Important side effects:** Nausea, vomiting, nervousness, anxiety. Use with caution on patients with history of

(continued)

Drug, Its Forms and Dosage Increments	Children and Adult Dosages and Instructions	Information and Important Side Effects
Syrup: 50 mg/5 mL 5 days - $	**Children >13 or adults:** 100 mg Q12H × 7 days. **Elderly:** Reduce dose to 100 mg Q24H	seizure disorder, renal or hepatic disease.
Zanamivir (Influenza A and B) (Relenza®) Pregnancy: C; Lactation: Unk **Rotadisk:** 5-mg blisters of powder for inhalation. 5 days - $$$	**Adults and Children >7 years:** 2 inhalations Q12H × 5 days.	**Food:** N/A **Important side effects:** Caution in patients with history of bronchospasm.

BRONCHOPULMONARY – Pertussis (*Bordetella pertussis*)

Drug, Its Forms and Dosage Increments	Children and Adult Dosages and Instructions	Information and Important Side Effects
<u>Erythromycin estolate or base</u>* Estolate salt recommended. (Ilosone®, E-mycin®, Ery-Tab®) Generics available Pregnancy: B; Lactation: Unsafe **Estolate:** **Tabs:** 500 mg **Caps:** 250 mg **Susp:** 125 mg/5 mL and 250 mg/5 mL **Oral Drops:** 100 mg/mL 250 mg/5 mL Q12H × 10 days - $ **Base:** **Tabs:** 250 mg, 333 mg, 500 mg	**Children:** 40-50 mg/kg/day **Estolate** (max 2 g/day) in two to four divided doses daily for 7-14 days. Erythromycin base dose is every 6 hours for 14 days. **Erythromycin Estolate** **250 mg/5 mL @ 40 mg/kg/day** 4-6 kg (10-15 lb) = ½ tsp (2.5 mL) Q12H 7-11 kg (16-25 lb) = 1 tsp (5 mL) Q12H 12-16 kg (26-35 lb) = 1½ tsp (7.5 mL) Q12H 17-25 kg (37-55 lb) = 2 tsp (10 mL) Q12H 26-37 kg (57-81 lb) = 2 tsp (10 mL) Q8H >38 kg (83 lb) = 1,000 mg Q12H	**Food:** May take with or without meals. Take with food if causes GI upset. **Important side effects:** GI upset, hepatitis.

Caps: 250 mg 500 mg PO Q6H × 10 days - $	**Adult:** Erythromycin estolate 500 mg PO four times daily for 7-14 days or Erythromycin base 500 mg PO four times daily for 14 days.	
Azithromycin* (Zithromax®) Pregnancy: B; Lactation: Unk **Tabs:** 250 mg and Z-Pak (500 mg × 1 day, then 250 mg daily × 4) **Oral Susp:** 100 mg/5 mL, 200 mg/5 mL 20 kg child - $$ Z-Pak - $$$	**Children ≥2 years:** 10-12 mg/kg/day (max 500 mg) PO once daily for 5-7 days. **100 mg/5 mL** 10 kg (22 lb) = 1 tsp (5 mL) PO once daily for 5-7 days. **200 mg/5 mL** 20 kg (44 lb) = 1 tsp (5 mL) Q24H 30 kg (66 lb) = 1½ tsp (7.5 mL) Q24H ≥40 kg (88 lb) = 2 tsp (10 mL) Q24H **Adolescent ≥16 years and Adult:** Dispense one Z-Pak.	**Food:** Oral suspension should be taken 1 hour before or 2 hours after food. Tablets may be taken without regard to food. **Important side effects:** Nausea, diarrhea, elevated LFTs.
Clarithromycin* (Biaxin, Biaxin XL®) Pregnancy: C; Lactation: Unk **Tabs:** 250 mg, 500 mg **Extended Release Tab (XL):** 500 mg **Oral Susp:** 125 mg/5 mL, 250 mg/5 mL 250 mg/5 mL Q12H × 10 days - $$ 500 mg PO Q12H × 10 days - $$$$	**Children ≥6 months:** 15 mg/kg/day (max 1 g/day) PO in divided doses twice daily for 5-7 days. **125 mg/tsp** 9 kg (20 lb) = ½ tsp (2.5 mL) Q12H 17 kg (37 lb) = 1 tsp (5 mL) Q12H **250 mg/tsp** 25 kg (55 lb) = ¾ tsp Q12H 33 kg (73 lb) = 1 tsp (5 mL) Q12H **Adult:** 500 mg PO twice daily for 7 days.	**Food:** Extended release tablet with food. Others without regard to food. **Important side effects:** Nausea, drug interactions.

(continued)

BRONCHOPULMONARY – Pertussis (*Bordetella pertussis*)

Drug, Its Forms and Dosage Increments	Children and Adult Dosages and Instructions	Information and Important Side Effects
Trimethoprim/Sulfamethoxazole* Considered second-line therapy. (Bactrim®, Septra®) Generics available Pregnancy: C; Lactation: Unsafe **Single Strength (SS) Tabs:** 80 mg/400 mg - >$ **Double Strength (DS) Tabs:** 160 mg/800 mg - >$ **Oral Susp:** 40 mg/200 mg per 5 mL - <$ - $	**Children ≥2 months:** 6-12 mg/kg/day TMP component (max 320 mg/day) in divided doses twice daily for 7-14 days. **40 mg/200 mg/5 mL @ 8 mg/kg/day** 10 kg (22 lb) = 1 tsp (5 mL) Q12H 20 kg (44 lb) = 2 tsp (10 mL) or 1 SS Tab Q12H 30 kg (66 lb) = 3 tsp (15 mL) or 1½ SS Tab Q12H 40 kg (88 lb) = 4 tsp (20 mL) or 2 SS Tabs or 1 DS Tab Q12H . **Adult:** 1 DS tablet PO twice daily for 14 days.	**Food:** May take without regard to food. Encourage fluids. **Important side effects:** Photosensitivity, rash.

BRONCHOPULMONARY – Pneumonia – Community-acquired Empiric therapy: Advanced generation macrolide, doxycycline or fluoroquinolone with good antipneumococcal activity.
(*Streptococcus pneumoniae, Mycoplasma pneumoniae, Haemophilus influenzae, Moraxella catarrhalis, Chlamydia pneumoniae, Legionella sp.*)

Drug, Its Forms and Dosage Increments	Children and Adult Dosages and Instructions	Information and Important Side Effects
Azithromycin* (Zithromax®) Pregnancy: B; Lactation: Unk **Tabs:** 250 mg and Z-Pak (500 mg × 1 day, then 250 mg daily × 4) **Oral Susp:** 100 mg/5 mL, 200 mg/5 mL	**Children ≥6 months:** 10 mg/kg/day (max 500 mg) once × 1 day, then 5 mg/kg/day (max 250 mg) once daily × 4 days. **100 mg/5 mL** 10 kg (22 lb) = 1 tsp (5 mL) once × 1 day, then ½ tsp (2.5 mL) daily for days 2-5.	**Food:** Oral suspension should be taken 1 hour before or 2 hours after food. Tablets may be taken without regard to food. **Important side effects:** Nausea, diarrhea, elevated LFTs.

20-kg child - $$ Z-Pak - $$$	**200 mg/5 mL** 20 kg (44 lb) = 1 tsp (5 mL) once × 1 day, then ½ tsp (2.5 mL) daily for days 2-5. .30 kg (66 lb) = 1½ tsp (7.5 mL) (2.5 mL) once × 1 day, then ¾ tsp daily for days 2-5. **Adult:** Dispense one Z-Pak.	
Clarithromycin* (Biaxin, Biaxin XL®) Pregnancy: C; Lactation: Unk **Tabs:** 250 mg, 500 mg **Extended Release Tab (XL):** 500 mg **Oral Susp:** 125 mg/5 mL, 250 mg/5 mL 250 mg/5 mL Q12H × 10 days - $$$ 500 mg PO Q12H × 10 days - $$$$	**Children ≥6 months:** 15 mg/kg/day (max 1 g/day) PO in divided doses twice daily for 7-10 days. **125 mg/5 mL** 9 kg (20 lb) = ½ tsp (2.5 mL) Q12H 17 kg (37 lb) = 1 tsp (5 mL) Q12H **250 mg/5 mL** 25 kg (55 lb) = ¾ tsp Q12H 33 kg (73 lb) = 1 tsp (5 mL) Q12H **Adult:** 500 mg PO twice daily or 1 gXL once daily for 7-10 days.	**Food:** Extended release tablet with food. Others without regard to food. **Important side effects:** Nausea, drug interactions.
Doxycycline* *For macrolide allergic patients.* *Not active vs. Legionella* (Vibramycin®) Generics available Pregnancy: D; Lactation: Unsafe **Caps:** 50 mg, 100 mg **Tabs:** 50 mg, 100 mg 100 mg PO Q12H × 10 days <$	**Adolescents ≥8 years or Adult:** 100 mg PO twice daily for 7-10 days.	**Food:** May take with food if GI upset occurs. Take 1 hour before or 2 hours after antacids, iron, milk, or other dairy products. Take with full glass of water to prevent esophagitis. **Important side effects:** Photosensitivity (use sunscreen), esophagitis. May discolor fingernails.

(continued)

Drug, Its Forms and Dosage Increments	Children and Adult Dosages and Instructions	Information and Important Side Effects
Erythromycin estolate or base* *In nonsmoker; not active vs. H. influenzae.* (Ilosone®, E-mycin®, Ery-Tab®) Generics available Pregnancy: B; Lactation: Unsafe **Estolate:** **Tabs:** 500 mg **Caps:** 250 mg **Susp:** 125 mg/5 mL and 250 mg/5 mL **Oral Drops:** 100 mg/mL 250 mg/5 mL Q12H × 10 days - $ **Base:** **Tabs:** 250 mg, 333 mg, 500 mg **Caps:** 250 mg 500 mg PO Q6H × 10 days - $	**Children:** 40 mg/kg/day estolate (max 2 g/day) in two to four divided doses daily for 7-10 days. **125 mg/5 mL @ 40 mg/kg/day** 3 kg (7 lb) = ½ tsp (2.5 mL) Q12H 6 kg (14 lb) = 1 tsp (5 mL) Q12H 9 kg (21 lb) = 1 tsp (5 mL) Q8H 13 kg (28 lb) = 2 tsp (10 mL) Q12H or 1 tsp (5 mL) PO Q6H **250 mg/5 mL @ 40 mg/kg/day** 13 kg (28 lb) = 1 tsp (5 mL) Q12H 19 kg (40 lb) = 1 tsp (5 mL) Q8H 25 kg (55 lb) = 1 tsp (5 mL) Q6H 37 kg (82 lb) = 2 tsp (10 mL) Q8H **Adult:** Erythromycin base or estolate 500 mg PO four times daily for 7-10 days.	**Food:** May take with or without meals. Take with food if causes GI upset. **Important side effects:** GI upset, hepatitis. **Note:** May cause greater GI upset than newer generation macrolides, such as azithromycin and clarithromycin.
Fluoroquinolones: Increased activity vs. above agents against drug-resistant *S. pneumoniae*. To help avoid developing resistance, consider reserving therapy with these agents to patients who have undergone unsuccessful therapy or are allergic or intolerant to above agents, or have documented drug-resistant *S. pneumoniae* (Penicillin MIC ≥4 μg/mL).		
Gatifloxacin* (Tequin®) Pregnancy: C; Lactation: Unsafe Tabs: 400 mg - $$$-$$$$	**Adult:** 400 mg PO Q24H for 7-10 days.	**Food:** May take with or without meals. Do not take within 4 hours of sucralfate, antacids, vitamins, or mineral products.

		Important side effects: Dizziness, photosensitivity, headache. **Reduce dose in severe renal disease (CrCl <40 mL/min).**
Levofloxacin* (Levaquin®) Pregnancy: C; Lactation: Unsafe **Tabs:** 250 mg, 500 mg - >$$$$	**Adult:** 500 mg PO once daily for 7-10 days.	**Food:** May take with or without meals. Do not take within 2 hours of antacids, magnesium, calcium supplements, zinc, aluminum, sucralfate, vitamins, or minerals (iron or zinc). **Important side effects:** Photosensitivity, dizziness. **Reduce dose in severe renal disease (CrCl <50 mL/min).**
Moxifloxacin* Avelox® Pregnancy: C; Lactation: Unk **Tabs:** 400 mg - >$$$$	**Adult:** 400 mg PO once daily for 7-14 days.	**Food:** May take without regard to food. Must take 4 hours before or 8 hours after sucralfate, antacids, aluminum, magnesium, calcium, zinc, iron, vitamins, or mineral supplements. **Important side effects:** Photosensitivity, dizziness, headache, insomnia, rash (may be severe), drug interactions.

Alternatives Beta-lactams not active against atypical organisms. High-dose amoxicillin for suspected pneumococcal pneumonia, but does not reliably cover *H. influenzae.*

Amoxicillin (Amoxil®) Generics available	**Children:** 80-90 mg/kg/day (max 1500 mg/day) in divided doses three times daily for 10-14 days.	**Food:** May take with or without meals.

(continued)

Drug, Its Forms and Dosage Increments	Children and Adult Dosages and Instructions	Information and Important Side Effects
Pregnancy: B; Lactation: Unsafe **Caps:** 250 mg, 500 mg - <$ **Tabs:** 500 mg, 875 mg - <$ **Chewable Tabs:** 125 mg, 200 mg, 250 mg, 400 mg - <$ **Suspension:** 125 mg/5 mL, 250 mg/5 mL, 400 mg/5 mL - $$ **Oral drops:** 50 mg/mL	**250 mg/5 mL at 80 mg/kg/day** 8 kg (18 lb) = 1 tsp (5 mL) Q8H 13 kg (29 lb) = 1½ tsp (7.5 mL) Q8H 17 kg (37 lb) = 2 tsp (10 mL) Q8H 21 kg (46 lb) = 2½ tsp (12.5 mL) (NTE 500 mg) Q8H 25 kg (55 lb) = 3 tsp (15 mL) (NTE 500 mg) Q8H **Adult:** 1 g PO three times daily for 7-10 days.	**Important side effects:** Diarrhea and nausea. May cause nonallergic maculopapular rash. **Reduce dose if renal disease (CrCl <30 mL/min).**
Amoxicillin/clavulanate (Augmentin®) Pregnancy: B; Lactation: Unk **Q12H Formulations:** **Tabs:** 500 mg/125 mg, 875 mg/125 mg - >$$$$	**Adult:** 875 mg/125 mg Q12H × 10-14 days.	**Food:** Take with meals to reduce diarrhea. **Side effects:** Diarrhea (take with food). May cause nonallergic amoxicillin rash. Nausea, rash. **Use with caution in hepatic disease.** **Reduce dose if renal disease (CrCl <30 mL/min).**
Cefpodoxime Vantin® Pregnancy: B; Lactation: Unk **Tabs:** 100 mg - $3.05 - $$-$$$ 200 mg - $4.03 - $$$-$$$ **Granules for Oral Suspension:** 50 mg/5 mL (50 mL, 75 mL, 100 mL) 100 mL - $$	**Children ≥5 months to 12 years:** 10 mg/kg/day in one or two divided doses (max 400 mg/day) for 10-14 days. **50 mg/tsp @ 10 mg/kg/day** 10 kg (22 lb) = 1 tsp (5 mL) Q12H or 2 tsp (10 mL) Q24H 15 kg (33 lb) = 1½ tsp (7.5 mL) Q12H or 3 tsp (15 mL) Q24H	**Food:** Take tablet with food. Suspension may be taken without regard to food. **Important side effects:** Nausea, vomiting, rash, diarrhea, elevated LFTs.

100 mg/5 mL (50 ml, 75 mL, 100 mL)
100 mL - $$$

100 mg/tsp @10 mg/kg/day
15 kg (33 lb) = ¾ tsp Q12H or 1½ tsp (7.5 mL) Q24H
20 kg (44 lb) = 1 tsp (5 mL) Q12H
30 kg (66 lb) = 1½ tsp (7.5 mL) Q12H or 3 tsp (15 mL) Q24H
40 kg (88 lb) = Use adult dose.
≥12 years to Adult: 200-400 mg twice daily for 7-14 days.

Cefuroxime axetil
(Ceftin®)
Pregnancy: B; Lactation: Unsafe
Tabs: 125 mg, 250 mg, 500 mg
Oral Susp: 125 mg/5 mL, 250 mg/5 mL
125 mg/5 mL Q12H × 10 days - $$
250 mg PO Q12H × 10 days - $$$$

Children >3 months to 12 years:
30 mg/kg/day (max 1 g/day) in divided doses twice daily for 7-14 days.
125 mg/5 mL @ 30 mg/kg/day
8 kg (18 lb) = 1 tsp (5 mL) (5 mL) Q12H
12.5 kg (27 lb) = 1½ tsp (7.5 mL) Q12H
17 kg (37 lb) = 2 tsp (10 mL) Q12H
25 kg (55 lb) = 3 tsp (15 mL) Q12H
33 kg (73 lb) = Use adult dose.
Children ≥13 years or Adult: 500 mg PO twice daily for 7-10 days.

Food: Take suspension with food. Tablets may be taken without regard to food.
Important side effects: Nausea, vomiting, rash.
Reduce dose if renal disease (CrCl <30 mL/min).

SKIN – Simple Abscess, Furuncle, Carbuncle, Folliculitis *(Staphylococcus aureus, Streptococcus sp.)*

Dicloxacillin
(Dynapen®)
Generics available
Pregnancy: B; Lactation: Unk
Caps: 125 mg, 250 mg, 500 mg

Children ≤40 kg: 25-50 mg/kg/day (max 2 g/day) in divided doses every 6 hours for 10-14 days.
62.5 mg/5 mL @ 25 mg/kg/day (double for 50 mg)

Food: Take 1 hour before or 2 hours after meals.
Important side effects: Bad taste, GI upset, vomiting, diarrhea.

(continued)

Drug, Its Forms and Dosage Increments	Children and Adult Dosages and Instructions	Information and Important Side Effects
Oral Susp: 62.5 mg/5 mL 200 mL - $ Adult 10-14 days - $	10 kg (22 lb) = 1 tsp (5 mL) Q6H 15 kg (33 lb) = 1½ tsp (7.5 mL) Q6H 20 kg (44 lb) = 2 tsp (10 mL) Q6H 40 kg (88 lb) = Use adult dose. **Children ≥40 kg and Adult:** 250-500 mg PO four times daily for 10-14 days.	
<u>**Cephalexin**</u> (Keflex®) Generics available Pregnancy: B; Lactation: Unk **Tabs:** 250 mg, 500 mg, 1 g **Caps:** 250 mg, 500 mg **Oral Susp:** 125 mg/5 mL, 250 mg/5 mL 250 mg/5 mL Q6H × 10 days - <$ 500 mg PO Q6H × 10 days - $	**Children:** 25-50 mg/kg/day (max 4 g/day) in divided doses two to four times daily for 10-14 days. **125 mg/5 mL @ 25 mg/kg/day** (double for 50 mg/kg) 10 kg (22 lb) = ½ tsp (2.5 mL) Q6H 15 kg (33 lb) = ¾ tsp Q6H **250 mg/5 mL @ 25 mg/kg/day** (double for 50 mg/kg) 20 kg (44 lb) = ½ tsp (2.5 mL) Q6H 40 kg (88 lb) = 1 tsp (5 mL) Q6H >40 kg = Use adult dose. **Adult:** 500 mg PO two to four times daily for 10-14 days.	**Food:** Take 1 hour before or 2 hours after meals. May take with food if GI upset occurs. **Important side effects:** GI upset, diarrhea. **Reduce dose if renal disease (CrCl <40 mL/min).**
Amoxicillin/clavulanate (Augmentin®) Pregnancy: B; Lactation: Unk	**Children:** 40-45 mg amoxicillin component/kg/day (max 1600 mg/day) in divided doses two or three times daily for 7-14 days.	**Food:** Take with food to reduce diarrhea. **Important side effects:** Diarrhea (common), nausea, rash.

Q12H Formulations:
Tabs: 500 mg/125 mg,
875 mg/125 mg - >$$$$
Chewable Tabs:
200 mg/28.5 mg, 400 mg/57 mg
Oral Susp: 200 mg/28.5 mg/5 mL,
400 mg/57 mg/5 mL

Q12H using 200 mg/5 mL susp @ 45 mg/kg/day
9 kg (20 lb) = 1 tsp (5 mL) Q12H
13 kg (29 lb) = 1½ tsp (7.5 mL) Q12H
18 kg (40 lb) = 2 tsp (10 mL) Q12H
Q12H using 400 mg/5 mL susp @ 45 mg/kg/day
18 kg (40 lb) = 1 tsp (5 mL) Q12H
27 kg (59 lb) = 1½ tsp (7.5 mL) Q12H
35 kg (77 lb) = 2 tsp (10 mL) Q12H
>40 kg = Use adult dose (max 875 mg Q12H)
Adult: 500-875 mg twice daily for 7-14 days.
Note: Q12H dosing may improve compliance compared to Q8H dosing.

Use with caution in hepatic disease. Reduce dose in renal disease (CrCl <30 mL/min).

Clindamycin*
A drug of choice for patients with penicillin or cephalosporin intolerance.
(Cleocin®)
Generics available
Pregnancy: B; Lactation: Unk
Caps: 75 mg, 150 mg, 300 mg
Oral Solution: 75 mg/5 mL
150 mg/10 mL Q8H × 10 days - $$$
300 mg PO Q6H × 10 days - $$

Children: Mild to Moderate: 10-15 mg/kg/day (max 1.8 g/day) PO in divided doses three or four times daily for 10-14 days.
Children: Severe: 16-25 mg/kg/day (max 1.8 g/day) in divided doses three or four times daily for 10-14 days.
75 mg/5 mL @ 10 mg/kg/day divided
10 kg (22 lb) = ½ tsp (2.5 mL) Q8H
20 kg (44 lb) = 1 tsp (5 mL) Q8H

Food: May take with or without meals. Take with full glass of water to prevent esophagitis.
Important side effects: Diarrhea (may be severe), nausea.
May cause severe colitis. Encourage patient to report severe, persistent, or bloody diarrhea.

(continued)

Drug, Its Forms and Dosage Increments	Children and Adult Dosages and Instructions	Information and Important Side Effects
	30 kg (66 lb) = 1½ tsp (7.5 mL) Q8H 40 kg (88 lb) = 2 tsp (10 mL) Q8H >40 kg = Use adult dose. **Adult: Mild to Moderate:** 150-300 mg PO three to four times daily for 10-14 days. **Adult: Severe:** 450 mg PO four times daily for 10-14 days.	
Erythromycin estolate or base* A drug of choice for patients with penicillin or cephalosporin intolerance (E-mycin®, Ilosone®) Generics available Pregnancy: B; Lactation: Unsafe **Estolate:** **Tabs:** 500 mg **Caps:** 250 mg **Susp:** 125 mg/5 mL and 250 mg/5 mL 250 mg/5 mL Q12H × 10 days - $ **Base:** **Tabs:** 250 mg, 333 mg, 500 mg **Caps:** 250 mg 500 mg PO Q6H × 10 days - $	**Children:** 20-40 mg/kg/day estolate (max 2 g/day) in two to four divided doses daily for 10-14 days. **125 mg/5 mL @ 20 mg/kg/day** 4-6 kg (10-15 lb) = ½ tsp (2.5 mL) Q12H 7-11 kg (16-25 lb) = 1 tsp (5 mL) Q12H 12-16 kg (26-35 lb) = 1½ tsp (7.5 mL) Q12H **250 mg/5 mL @ 20 mg/kg/day** 17-25 kg = 1 tsp (5 mL) Q12H 26-37 kg = 1½ tsp (7.5 mL) Q12H >38 kg = 500 mg Q12H **Adult:** Erythromycin base or estolate 500 mg PO four times daily for 10-14 days.	**Food:** May take with or without meals. Take with food if causes GI upset. **Important side effects:** GI upset, hepatitis.

SKIN – Bite Wound – Cat Bite (*Pasteurella multocida*, mixed flora) **Give tetanus prophylaxis.** Outpatient management with oral antimicrobial therapy may be appropriate for early, minor, wounds. Many patients, especially those with bite to the hand, face, or groin may require hospitalization and surgical (orthopaedic) consultation.

<u>**Amoxicillin/clavulanate**</u> (Augmentin®) Pregnancy: B; Lactation: Unk **Q12H Formulations:** **Tabs:** 500 mg/125 mg, 875 mg/125 mg **Chewable Tabs:** 200 mg/28.5 mg, 400 mg/57 mg **Oral Susp:** 200 mg/28.5 mg/5 mL, 400 mg/57 mg/5 mL Child - $$$ Adult - >$$$$	**Children:** 40-45 mg amoxicillin component/kg/day (max 1600 mg/day) in divided doses two or three times daily; reevaluate in 3-5 days to determine need for debridement and duration of therapy. **Q12H using 200 mg/5 mL susp @ 45 mg/kg/day** 9 kg (20 lb) = 1 tsp (5 mL) Q12H 13 kg (29 lb) = 1½ tsp (7.5 mL) Q12H 18 kg (40 lb) = 2 tsp (10 mL) Q12H **Q12H using 400 mg/5 mL susp @ 45 mg/kg/day** 18 kg (40 lb) = 1 tsp (5 mL) Q12H 27 kg (59 lb) = 1½ tsp (7.5 mL) Q12H 35 kg (77 lb) = 2 tsp (10 mL) Q12H >40 kg = Use adult dose (max 875 mg Q12H). **Adult:** 500-875 mg twice daily for 3-5 days. Note: Q12H dosing may improve compliance compared to Q8H dosing.	**Food:** Take with food to reduce diarrhea. **Important side effects:** Diarrhea (common), nausea, rash. **Use cautiously in hepatic disease.** **Reduce dose in renal disease (CrCl <30 mL/min).**
Cefuroxime axetil (Ceftin®) Pregnancy: B; Lactation: Unsafe	**Children >3 months to 12 years:** 30 mg/kg/day (max 1 g/day) in divided doses twice daily for 3-5 days.	**Food:** Take suspension with food. Tablets may be taken without regard to food.

(continued)

Drug, Its Forms and Dosage Increments	Children and Adult Dosages and Instructions	Information and Important Side Effects
Tabs: 125 mg, 250 mg, 500 mg **Oral Susp:** 125 mg/5 mL, 250 mg/5 mL 125 mg/5 mL Q12H × 10 days - $$ 250 mg PO Q12H × 10 days - $$$$	**125 mg/5 mL @ 30 mg/kg/day** 8 kg (18 lb) = 1 tsp (5 mL) (5 mL) Q12H 12.5 kg (27 lb) = 1½ tsp (7.5 mL) Q12H 17 kg (37 lb) = 2 tsp (10 mL) Q12H 25 kg (55 lb) = 3 tsp (15 mL) Q12H 33 kg (73 lb) = Use adult dose. **Children ≥13 years or Adult:** 500 mg PO twice daily for 3-5 days.	**Important side effects:** Nausea, vomiting, rash. **Reduce dose if renal disease (CrCl <30 mL/min).**
Doxycycline* **An alternative for patients with beta-lactam intolerance.** (Vibramycin®) Generics available Pregnancy: D; Lactation: Unsafe **Caps:** 50 mg, 100 mg - <$ **Tabs:** 50 mg, 100 mg - <$	**Children ≥8 years and Adult:** 100 mg PO twice daily for 3-5 days.	**Food:** May take with food if GI upset occurs. Take 1 hour before or 2 hours after antacids, iron, milk, or other dairy products. Take with full glass of water to prevent esophagitis. **Important side effects:** Photosensitivity, (use sunscreen), esophagitis. May discolor fingernails.

SKIN – Bite Wound – Dog Bite (*Pasteurella multocida, P. canis, Viridans streptococci, Staphylococcus aureus,* anaerobes) **Give tetanus prophylaxis.** Evaluate need for rabies prophylaxis. Outpatient management with oral antimicrobial therapy may be appropriate for early, minor, wounds. Many patients, especially those with bite to the hand, face, or groin may require hospitalization and surgical (orthopaedic) consultation.

Drug, Its Forms and Dosage Increments	Children and Adult Dosages and Instructions	Information and Important Side Effects
Amoxicillin/clavulanate (Augmentin®) Pregnancy: B; Lactation: Unk	**Children:** 40-45 mg amoxicillin component/kg/day (max 1600 mg/day) in divided doses two or three times daily; reevaluate in 3-5 days to determine	**Food:** Take with food to reduce diarrhea. **Important side effects:** Diarrhea (common), nausea, rash.

Q12H Formulations:
Tabs: 500 mg/125 mg, 875 mg/125 mg
Chewable Tabs:
200 mg/28.5 mg, 400 mg/57 mg
Oral Susp:
200 mg/28.5 mg/5 mL,
400 mg/57 mg/5 mL
Child - $$$ Adult - >$$$$

need for debridement and duration of therapy.

Q12H using 200 mg/5 mL susp @ 45 mg/kg/day
9 kg (20 lb) = 1 tsp (5 mL) Q12H
13 kg (29 lb) = 1½ tsp (7.5 mL) Q12H
18 kg (40 lb) = 2 tsp (10 mL) Q12H

Q12H using 400 mg/5 mL susp @ 45 mg/kg/day
18 kg (40 lb) = 1 tsp (5 mL) Q12H
27 kg (59 lb) = 1½ tsp (7.5 mL) Q12H
35 kg (77 lb) = 2 tsp (10 mL) Q12H
>40 kg = Use adult dose (max 875 mg Q12H).

Adult: 500-875 mg twice daily for 3-5 days.

Use cautiously in hepatic disease. Reduce dose in renal disease (CrCl <30 mL/min).

Clindamycin*
An alternative for patients with beta-lactam intolerance.
(Cleocin®
Generics available
Pregnancy: B; Lactation: Unk
Caps: 75 mg, 150 mg, 300 mg - $$$
Oral Solution: 75 mg/5 mL
Must administer clindamycin with a fluoroquinolone (adults) or trimethoprim/sulfamethoxazole (children).

Children: 10-20 mg/kg/day (max 1200 mg/day) in divided doses three or four times daily for 3-5 days.

75 mg/5 mL @ 10 mg/kg/day divided Q8H
10 kg (22 lb) = ½ tsp (2.5 mL) Q8H
20 kg (44 lb) = 1 tsp (5 mL) Q8H
30 kg (66 lb) = 1½ tsp (2.5 mL) (7.5 mL) Q8H
40 kg (88 lb) = 2 tsp (10 mL) Q8H
50 kg (110 lb) = 300 mg PO Q8H
≥60 kg and Adult: 300 mg PO four times daily for 3-5 days.

Food: May take with or without meals. Take with full glass of water to prevent esophagitis.
Important side effects: Diarrhea (may be severe), nausea.

(continued)

Drug, Its Forms and Dosage Increments	Children and Adult Dosages and Instructions	Information and Important Side Effects
Ciprofloxacin* (Cipro®) Pregnancy: C; Lactation: Unsafe **Tabs:** 250 mg, 500 mg, 750 mg - >$$$$ **Use fluoroquinolone in conjunction with clindamycin in adults with beta-lactam intolerance.**	**≥18 years:** 500 mg PO twice daily for 3-5 days.	**Food:** Take on empty stomach 1 hour before or 2 hours after a meal. May take with food if it causes GI upset, but avoid large amounts of dairy products. May take 2 hours before or 6 hours after sucralfate, antacids, aluminum, magnesium, calcium, zinc, iron, vitamins, or mineral supplements. **Important side effects:** Photosensitivity, dizziness. **Reduce dose in renal disease (CrCl <50 mL/min).**
Trimethoprim/Sulfamethoxazole* (Bactrim®, Septra®) Generics available Pregnancy: C; Lactation: Unsafe **Single Strength (SS)** **Tabs:** 80 mg/400 mg - <$ **Double Strength (DS)** **Tabs:** 160 mg/800 mg - <$ **Oral Susp:** 40 mg/200 mg per 5 mL - $ **Use in conjunction with clindamycin in persons with beta-lactam intolerance.**	**Children ≥2 months:** 6-12 mg/kg/day TMP component (max 320 mg/day) in divided doses twice daily for 3-5 days. **40 mg/200 mg/5 mL** 10 kg (22 lb) = 1 tsp (5 mL) Q12H . 20 kg (44 lb) = 2 tsp (10 mL) or 1 SS Tab Q12H 30 kg (66 lb) = 3 tsp (15 mL) or 1½ SS Tab Q12H 40 kg (88 lb) = 4 tsp (20 mL) or 2 SS Tabs **or** 1 DS Tab Q12H for 10 days. **Adult:** 1 DS tablet PO twice daily for 3-5 days.	**Food:** May take without regard to food. Encourage fluids. **Important side effects:** Photosensitivity, rash. **Reduce dose in renal disease (CrCl <30 mL/min).**

SKIN – Bite Wound – Human Bite (*Viridans streptococci, Streptococcus epidermidis, Staphylococcus aureus, Corynebacterium, Eikenella*, anaerobes) Outpatient management with oral antimicrobial therapy may be appropriate for early, minor, wounds. Many patients, especially those with bite to the hand, face, or groin may require hospitalization and surgical (orthopaedic) consultation.

Amoxicillin/clavulanate
(Augmentin®)
Pregnancy: B; Lactation: Unk
Q12H Formulations:
Tabs: 500 mg/125 mg, 875 mg/125 mg
Chewable Tabs:
200 mg/28.5 mg, 400 mg/57 mg
Oral Susp:
200 mg/28.5 mg/5 mL,
400 mg/57 mg/5 mL
Child - $$$ Adult - >$$$$.

Children: 40-45 mg amoxicillin component/kg/day (max 1600 mg/day) in divided doses two or three times daily; reevaluate in 3-5 days to determine need for debridement and duration of therapy.

Q12H using 200 mg/5 mL susp @ 45 mg/kg/day
9 kg (20 lb) = 1 tsp (5 mL) Q12H
13 kg (29 lb) = 1½ tsp (7.5 mL) Q12H
18 kg (40 lb) = 2 tsp (10 mL) Q12H

Q12H using 400 mg/5 mL susp @ 45 mg/kg/day
18 kg (40 lb) = 1 tsp (5 mL) Q12H
27 kg (59 lb) = 1½ tsp (7.5 mL) Q12H
35 kg (77 lb) = 2 tsp (10 mL) Q12H
>40 kg = Use adult dose (max 875 mg Q12H).

Adult: 500-875 mg twice daily for 3-5 days.

Food: Take with food to reduce diarrhea.
Important side effects: Diarrhea (common), nausea, rash.
Use with caution in hepatic disease.
Reduce dose in renal disease (CrCl <30 mL/min).

(continued)

Drug, Its Forms and Dosage Increments	Children and Adult Dosages and Instructions	Information and Important Side Effects
Clindamycin* **An alternative for patients with beta-lactam intolerance.** (Cleocin®) Generics available Pregnancy: B; Lactation: Unk **Caps:** 75 mg, 150 mg, 300 mg **Oral Sol:** 75 mg/5 mL **Must administer clindamycin with a fluoroquinolone (adults) or trimethoprim/sulfamethoxazole (children).**	**Children:** 10-20 mg/kg/day (max 1200 mg/day) in divided doses three or four times daily for 3-5 days. **75 mg/5 m @ 10 mg/kg/day divided Q8H** 10 kg (22 lb) = ½ tsp (2.5 mL) Q8H 20 kg (44 lb) = 1 tsp (5 mL) Q8H 30 kg (66 lb) = 1½ tsp (7.5 mL) Q8H 40 kg (88 lb) = 2 tsp (10 mL) Q8H 50 kg (110 lb) = 300 mg PO Q8H **≥60 kg and Adult:** 300 mg PO four times daily for 3-5 days.	**Food:** May take with or without meals. Take with full glass of water to prevent esophagitis. **Important side effects:** Diarrhea, may be severe. Nausea. ***May cause severe colitis.** Encourage patient to report severe, persistent, or bloody diarrhea.
Ciprofloxacin* (Cipro®) Pregnancy: C; Lactation: Unsafe **Tabs:** 250 mg, 500 mg **Use fluoroquinolone in conjunction with clindamycin in adults with beta-lactam intolerance.**	**≥18 years:** 500 mg PO twice daily; reevaluate in 3-5 days to determine need for debridement and duration of therapy.	**Food:** Take on empty stomach 1 hour before or 2 hours after a meal. May take with food if it causes GI upset, but avoid large amounts of dairy products. May take 2 hours before or 6 hours after sucralfate, antacids, aluminum, magnesium, calcium, zinc, iron, vitamins, or mineral supplements. **Important side effects:** Photosensitivity, dizziness. **Reduce dose in renal disease (CrCl <50 mL/min).**

Trimethoprim/Sulfamethoxazole* (Bactrim®, Septra®) Generics available Pregnancy: C; Lactation: Unsafe **Single Strength (SS) Tabs:** 80 mg/400 mg - <$ **Double Strength (DS) Tabs:** 160 mg/800 mg - <$ **Oral Susp:** 40 mg/200 mg per 5 mL - $ **Use in conjunction with clindamycin in persons with beta-lactam intolerance.**	**Children ≥2 months:** 6-12 mg/kg/day TMP component (max 320 mg/day) in divided doses twice daily for 3-5 days. **40 mg/200 mg/5 mL** 10 kg (22 lb) = 1 tsp (5 mL) Q12H 20 kg (44 lb) = 2 tsp (10 mL) or 1 SS Tab Q12H 30 kg (66 lb) = 3 tsp (15 mL) or 1½ SS Tab Q12H 40 kg (88 lb) = 4 tsp (20 mL) or 2 SS Tabs or 1 DS Q12H **Adult:** 1 DS tablet twice daily for 3-5 days.	**Food:** May take without regard to food. Encourage fluids. **Important side effects:** Photosensitivity, rash. **Reduce dose in renal disease (CrCl <30 mL/min).**

SKIN – Candidiasis (*Candida albicans*)

Nystatin* (Mycostatin®, Nilstat®) Generics available Pregnancy: B; Lactation: Safe **Cream 100,000 U/g:** 15 g, 30 g **Ointment 100,000 U/g:** 15 g, 30 g	**Adult:** Massage into affected area after washing and drying twice daily until all signs of infection are resolved.	**Important side effects:** Well tolerated. If irritation occurs, discontinue.

SKIN – Cat-Scratch (*Bartonella henselae*) Benefit of antimicrobial therapy in immunocompetent persons is not clearly established. Disease is generally self-limited.

Azithromycin* (Zithromax®) Pregnancy: B; Lactation: Unk	**Children ≥6 months:** 10 mg/kg/day (max 500 mg) once daily × 1 day, then 5 mg/kg/day (max 250 mg) once daily × 4 days	**Important side effects:** Palpitation, chest pain, jaundice.

(continued)

Drug, Its Forms and Dosage Increments	Children and Adult Dosages and Instructions	Information and Important Side Effects
Tabs: 250 mg and Z-Pak (500 mg × 1 day, then 250 mg daily × 4) **Oral Susp:** 100 mg/5 mL, 200 mg/5 mL 20-kg child - $$ Z-Pak - $$$	**100 mg/5 mL** 10 kg (22 lb) = 1 tsp (5 mL)/day × 1 day, then ½ tsp (2.5 mL) daily for days 2-5. **200 mg/5 mL** 20 kg (44 lb) = 1 tsp (5 mL)/day × 1 day, then ½ tsp (2.5 mL) daily for days 2-5. 30 kg (66 lb) = 1.5 tsp/day × 1 day, then ¾ tsp daily for days 2-5. **Adult:** Dispense one Z-Pak.	**Food:** Oral suspension and capsules should be taken 1 hour before or 2 hours after food. Tablets may be taken without regard to food.
Ciprofloxacin* (Cipro®) Pregnancy: C; Lactation: Unsafe **Tabs:** 250 mg, 500 mg, 750 mg - >$$$$	**Adult:** 500 mg PO twice daily for 10-14 days.	**Food:** Take on empty stomach 1 hour before or 2 hours after a meal. May take with food if it causes GI upset, but avoid large amounts of dairy products. May take 2 hours before or 6 hours after sucralfate, antacids, aluminum, magnesium, calcium, zinc, iron, vitamins, or mineral supplements. **Important side effects:** Photosensitivity, dizziness. **Reduce dose in renal disease (CrCl <50 mL/min).**
SKIN – Cellulitis – Mild (*Staphylococcus aureus*, Group A *Streptococcus*)		
Cephalexin (Keflex®) Generics available	**Children:** 25-100 mg/kg/day (max 4 g/day) in divided doses three or four times daily for 10-14 days.	**Food:** May take with food if GI upset occurs.

<table>
<tr><td>Pregnancy: B; Lactation: Unk
Tabs: 250 mg, 500 mg, 1 g
Caps: 250 mg, 500 mg
Oral Susp: 125 mg/5 mL, 250 mg/5 mL
250 mg/5 mL Q6H × 10 days - <$
500 mg PO Q6H × 10 days - $</td><td>**125 mg/5 mL @ 25 mg/kg/day** (double for 50 mg/kg)
10 kg (22 lb) = ½ tsp (2.5 mL) Q6H
15 kg (33 lb) = ¾ tsp Q6H
20 kg (44 lb) = 1 tsp (5 mL) Q6H
250 mg/5 mL @ 25 mg/kg/day (double for 50 mg/kg)
20 kg (44 lb) = ½ tsp (2.5 mL) Q6H
40 kg (88 lb) = 1 tsp (5 mL) Q6H
>40 kg = Use adult dose.
Adult: 500 mg PO four times daily for 10-14 days.</td><td>**Important side effects:** GI upset, diarrhea.
Reduce dose in renal disease (CrCl <40 mL/min).</td></tr>
<tr><td><u>**Dicloxacillin**</u>
(Dynapen®)
Generics available
Pregnancy: B; Lactation: Unk
Caps: 125 mg, 250 mg, 500 mg
Oral Susp: 62.5 mg/5 mL, 200 mL - $
Adult 10-14 days - $</td><td>**Children ≤40 kg:** 25-50 mg/kg/day (max 2 g/day) in divided doses every 6 hours for 10-14 days.
62.5 mg/5 mL @ 25 mg/kg/day (double for 50 mg)
10 kg (22 lb) = 1 tsp (5 mL) Q6H
15 kg (33 lb) = 1½ tsp (7.5 mL) Q6H
20 kg (44 lb) = 2 tsp (10 mL) Q6H
40 kg (88 lb) = Use adult dose.
Children ≥40 kg and Adult: 250-500 mg PO four times daily for 10-14 days.</td><td>**Food:** Take 1 hour before or 2 hours after meals.
Important side effects: Bad taste, GI upset; may reduce efficacy of oral contraceptives.</td></tr>
<tr><td>**Erythromycin estolate or base***
An alternative for patients with beta-lactam intolerance.</td><td>**Children:** 30-50 mg/kg/day estolate (max 2 g/day) in two to four divided doses a day for 10-14 days.</td><td>**Food:** May take with or without meals. Take with food if causes GI upset.</td></tr>
</table>

(continued)

Drug, Its Forms and Dosage Increments	Children and Adult Dosages and Instructions	Information and Important Side Effects
(E-mycin®, Ilosone®) Generics available Pregnancy: B; Lactation: Unsafe **Estolate:** **Tabs:** 500 mg **Caps:** 250 mg **Oral Susp:** 125 mg/5 mL, 250 mg/5 mL 250 mg/5 mL Q12H × 10 days - $ **Base:** **Tabs:** 250 mg, 333 mg, 500 mg **Caps:** 250 mg 500 mg PO Q6H × 10 days - $	**125 mg/5 mL @ 30 mg/kg/day** 4 kg (10 lb) = ½ tsp (2.5 mL) Q12H 5-8 kg (11-18 lb) = 1 tsp (5 mL) Q12H 9-12 kg (20-26 lb) = 1 tsp (5 mL) Q8H 13-16 kg (29-35 lb) = 1 tsp (5 mL) Q6H or 2 tsp (10 mL) Q12H **250 mg/5 mL @ 30 mg/kg/day** 13-16 kg (29-35 lb) = 1 tsp (5 mL) Q12H 17-25 kg (37-55 lb) = 1½ tsp (7.5 mL) Q12H or 1 tsp (5 mL) Q8H 26-33 kg (57-72 lb) = 250 mg Q6H or 500 mg Q12H 30-50 kg (66-110 lb) = 500 mg Q8H **Adult:** Erythromycin base or estolate 500 mg PO four times daily for 10-14 days.	**Important side effects:** GI upset, hepatitis.
Levofloxacin* (Levaquin®) Pregnancy: C; Lactation: Unsafe **Tabs:** 250 mg, 500 mg - $$$->$$$$	**Adult:** 500 mg PO once daily for 7-14 days.	**Food:** May take with or without meals. Do not take within 2 hours of antacids, magnesium, calcium supplements, zinc, aluminum, sucralfate, vitamins, or minerals (iron or zinc). **Important side effects:**Photosensitivity, dizziness. **Reduce dose in renal disease (CrCl <50 mL/min).**

SKIN – Cellulitis – Severe (Admit for IV antibiotics or consider outpatient parenteral therapy when appropriate & available).

SKIN – Diabetic Foot Mild-Moderate (*Staphylococcus aureus*, beta-hemolytic streptococci, gram negatives, anaerobes)
Non–limb-threatening infections may be treated with oral antibiotics in an outpatient setting. More severe infections, or those in an ischemic limb, require surgical consultation and often intravenous therapy.

Drug	Dosing	Comments
Cephalexin (Keflex®) Generics available Pregnancy: B; Lactation: Unk **Tabs:** 250 mg, 500 mg, 1 g **Caps:** 250 mg, 500 mg 500 mg PO Q6H × 14 days - $	**Adult:** 500 mg PO four times daily for 14 days.	**Food:** May take with food if GI upset occurs. **Important side effects:** GI upset, diarrhea. **Reduce dose in renal disease (CrCl <40 mL/min).**
Clindamycin* (Cleocin®) Generics available Pregnancy: B; Lactation: Unk **Caps:** 75 mg, 150 mg, 300 mg 300 mg PO Q6H × 14 days - $$$	**Adult:** 300 mg PO four times daily for 14 days.	**Food:** May take with or without meals. Take with full glass of water to prevent esophagitis. **Important side effects:** Diarrhea (may be severe), nausea. ***May cause severe colitis.** Encourage patient to report severe, persistent, or bloody diarrhea.
Amoxicillin/clavulanate (Augmentin®) Pregnancy: B; Lactation: Unk	**Adult:** 500-875 mg twice daily for 14 days. Note: Q12H dosing may improve compliance compared to Q8H dosing.	**Food:** Take with food to reduce diarrhea. **Important side effects:** Diarrhea (common), nausea, rash.

(continued)

Drug, Its Forms and Dosage Increments	Children and Adult Dosages and Instructions	Information and Important Side Effects
Q12H Formulations: **Tabs:** 500 mg/125 mg, 875 mg/125 mg Child - $$$ Adult - >$$$$		**Use cautiously in hepatic disease.** **Reduce dose in renal disease (CrCl <30 mL/min).**
Levofloxacin* **Alternative for failure of above drug.** (Levaquin®) Pregnancy: C; Lactation: Unsafe **Tabs:** 250 mg, 500 mg - >$$$$	**Adult:** 500 mg PO once daily for 14 days.	**Food:** May take with or without meals. Do not take within 2 hours of antacids, magnesium, calcium supplements, zinc, aluminum, sucralfate, vitamins, or minerals (iron or zinc). **Important side effects:** Photosensitivity, dizziness. **Reduce dose in renal disease (CrCl <50 mL/min).**
Trimethoprim/Sulfamethoxazole* (Bactrim®, Septra®) Generics available Pregnancy: C; Lactation: Unsafe **Single Strength (SS) Tabs** 80/400 - <$ **Double Strength (DS) Tabs** 160/800 - <$ **Susp** 40/200 mg/5 Ml - $	**Adult:** 1 DS Tab Q12H for 10-14 days.	**Food:** May take without regard to food. Encourage fluids. **Important side effects:** Photosensitivity, rash. **Reduce dose in renal disease (CrCl <30 mL/min).**

SKIN – Erysipelas, Mild to Moderate, Nondiabetic Person (Group A *Streptococcus, occasionally other Streptococcus sp., Staphylococcus aureus*)

Drug, Its Forms and Dosage Increments	Children and Adult Dosages and Instructions	Information and Important Side Effects
Penicillin V Potassium **A drug of choice, especially if staph is unlikely.**	**Children <12 years:** 25-50 mg/kg/day (max 2 g/day) PO in divided doses Q6H for 10 days.	**Food:** Take 1 hour before or 2 hours after meals. May take with food if GI upset occurs.

(Pen Vee K®) Generics available Pregnancy: B; Lactation: Unsafe **Tabs:** 125 mg, 250 mg, 500 mg **Oral Susp:** 125 mg/5 mL, 250 mg/5 mL 250 mg/5 mL Q6H × 10 days <$ 500 mg PO Q8H × 10 days <$	**125 mg/5 mL @ 25 mg/kg/day** 10 kg (22 lb) = ½ tsp (2.5 mL) Q6H 15 kg (33 lb) = ¾ tsp Q6H 20 kg (44 lb) = 1 tsp (5 mL) Q6H >20 kg (44 lb) = Use adult dose. **250 mg/5 mL @ 50 mg/kg/day** 10 kg (22 lb) = ½ tsp (2.5 mL) Q6H 15 kg (33 lb) = ¾ tsp Q6H 20 kg (44 lb) = 1 tsp (5 mL) Q6H >20 kg (44 lb) = Use adult dose. **Children ≥12 years and Adult:** 500 mg PO Q6H for 10-14 days.	**Important side effects:** Nausea, rash. Use with caution if history of seizure disorder.
Cephalexin (Keflex®) Generics available Pregnancy: B; Lactation: Unk **Tabs:** 250 mg, 500 mg, 1 g **Caps:** 250 mg, 500 mg **Oral Susp:** 125 mg/5 mL, 250 mg/5 mL 250 mg/5 mL Q6H × 10 days - <$ 500 mg PO Q6H × 10 days - $	**Children:** 25-100 mg/kg/day (max 4 g/day) PO in divided doses three or four times daily for 10-14 days. **125 mg/5 mL @ 25 mg/kg/day** (double for 50 mg/kg) 10 kg (22 lb) = ½ tsp (2.5 mL) Q6H 15 kg (33 lb) = ¾ tsp Q6H 20 kg (44 lb) = 1 tsp (5 mL) Q6H **250 mg/5 mL @ 25 mg/kg/day** (double for 50 mg/kg) 20 kg (44 lb) = ½ tsp (2.5 mL) Q6H 40 kg (88 lb) = 1 tsp (5 mL) Q6H >40 kg = Use adult dose. **Adult:** 500 mg PO four times daily for 10-14 days.	**Food:** May take with food if GI upset occurs. **Important side effects:** GI upset, diarrhea. **Reduce dose in renal disease (CrCl <40 mL/min).**

(continued)

Drug, Its Forms and Dosage Increments	Children and Adult Dosages and Instructions	Information and Important Side Effects
<u>Dicloxacillin</u> **A drug of choice, especially if staph is suspected.** (Dynapen®) Generics available Pregnancy: B; Lactation: Unk **Caps:** 125 mg, 250 mg, 500 mg **Oral Susp:** 62.5 mg/5 mL, 200 mL - $ Adult 10-14 days - $	**Children ≤40 kg:** 25-50 mg/kg/day (max 2 g/day) in divided doses every 6 hours for 10-14 days. **62.5 mg/5 mL @ 25 mg/kg/day** (double for 50 mg) 10 kg (22 lb) = 1 tsp (5 mL) Q6H 15 kg (33 lb) = 1½ tsp (7.5 mL) Q6H 20 kg (44 lb) = 2 tsp (10 mL) Q6H 40 kg (88 lb) = Use adult dose. **Children ≥40 kg and Adult:** 250-500 mg PO four times daily for 10-14 days.	**Food:** Take 1 hour before or 2 hours after meals. **Important side effects:** Bad taste, GI upset.
Erythromycin estolate or base* **An alternative for patients with beta-lactam intolerance.** (E-mycin®, Ilosone®) Generics available Pregnancy: B; Lactation: Unsafe **Estolate:** **Tabs:** 500 mg **Caps:** 250 mg **Oral Susp:** 125 mg/5 mL, 250 mg/5 mL 250 mg/5 mL Q12H × 10 days - $ **Base:** **Tabs:** 250 mg, 333 mg, 500 mg	**Children:** 30-50 mg/kg/day estolate (max 2 g/day) in two to four divided doses daily for 10-14 days. **125 mg/5 mL @ 30 mg/kg/day** 4 kg (10 lb) = ½ tsp (2.5 mL) Q12H 5-8 kg (11-18 lb) = 1 tsp (5 mL) Q12H 9-12 kg (20-26 lb) = 1 tsp (5 mL) Q8H 13-16 kg (29-35 lb) = 1 tsp (5 mL) Q6H or 2 tsp (10 mL) Q12H **250 mg/5 mL @ 30 mg/kg/day** 13-16 kg (29-35 lb) = 1 tsp (5 mL) Q12H 17-25 kg (37-55 lb) = 1½ tsp (7.5 mL) Q12H or 1 tsp (5 mL) Q8H	**Food:** May take with or without meals. Take with food if causes GI upset. **Important side effects:** GI upset, hepatitis.

Caps: 250 mg 500 mg PO Q6H × 10 days - $	26-33 kg (57-72 lb) = 250 mg Q6H or 500 mg Q12H 30-50 kg (66-110 lb) = 500 mg Q8H **Adult:** Erythromycin base or estolate 500 mg PO four times daily for 10-14 days.	

SKIN – Erysipelas – Severe, Nondiabetic Person (Group A *Streptococcus*, occasionally other *Streptococcus sp.*, *Staphylococcus aureus*) Initiate therapy in hospital with parenteral antimicrobials.

SKIN – Herpes Zoster, Varicella (Shingles) (*Varicella zoster*)
Note: If patient >50 years may benefit from prednisone for pain control.

Acyclovir* (Zovirax®) Pregnancy: C; Lactation: Safe **Caps:** 200 mg **Tabs:** 400 mg, 800 mg - $$-$$$ **Oral Susp:** 200 mg/5 mL - >$$$$	**Children 2-16 years:** 80 mg/kg/day (max 4 g/day) PO in divided doses four or five times daily for 7-10 days. **Adults:** 800 mg PO five times daily for 7-10 days.	**Food:** May be taken without regard to food. Encourage fluids. **Important side effects:** Headache, dizziness, nausea, seizures, bone-marrow suppression, nephrotoxicity. **Reduce dose in renal disease (CrCl <25 mL/min).**
Famciclovir* (Famvir®) Pregnancy: B; Lactation: Unsafe **Tabs:** 125 mg, 250 mg, 500 mg - >$$$$	**Children: N/A** **Adult:** 500 mg PO every 8 hours for 7 days.	**Food:** May take without regard to food. **Important side effects:** Nausea, headache, dizziness. **Reduce dose in renal disease (CrCl <60 mL/min).**
Valacyclovir* (Valtrex®) Pregnancy: B; Lactation: Unk	**Children: N/A** **Adult:** 1,000 mg PO three times daily for 7 days.	**Food:** May take without regard to food. **Important side effects:** Nausea, headache, dizziness.

(continued)

Drug, Its Forms and Dosage Increments	Children and Adult Dosages and Instructions	Information and Important Side Effects
Tabs: 500 mg, 1,000 mg - >$$$$		**Reduce dose in renal disease (CrCl <50 mL/min).**

SKIN – Impetigo – Mild, Nonbullous (Group A *Streptococcus, Staphylococcus aureus*)

Drug, Its Forms and Dosage Increments	Children and Adult Dosages and Instructions	Information and Important Side Effects
Mupirocin* (Bactroban®) Pregnancy: B; Lactation: Unk **Ointment 2%:** 15-g and 30-g tubes	**Children and Adult:** Apply to lesions three times daily for 5-10 days.	**Important side effects:** Burning, stinging, itching. Avoid contact with eye(s).
Cephalexin (Keflex®) Generics available Pregnancy: B; Lactation: Unk **Tabs:** 250 mg, 500 mg, 1 g **Caps:** 250 mg, 500 mg **Oral Susp:** 125 mg/5 mL, 250 mg/5 mL 250 mg/5 mL Q6H × 10 days - <$ 500 mg PO Q6H × 10 days - $	**Children**: 25-50 mg/kg/day (max 4 g/day) in divided doses two to four times daily for 10-14 days. **125 mg/5 mL @ 25 mg/kg/day** (double for 50 mg/kg) 10 kg (22 lb) = ½ tsp (2.5 mL) Q6H 15 kg (33 lb) = ¾ tsp Q6H **250 mg/5 mL @ 25 mg/kg/day** (double for 50 mg/kg) 20 kg (44 lb) = ½ tsp (2.5 mL) Q6H 40 kg (88 lb) = 1 tsp (5 mL) Q6H >40 kg = Use adult dose. **Adult:** 500 mg PO four times daily for 10-14 days.	**Food:** May take with food if GI upset occurs. **Important side effects:** GI upset, diarrhea. **Reduce dose in renal disease (CrCl <40 mL/min).**

Dicloxacillin (Dynapen®) Generics available Pregnancy: B; Lactation: Unk **Caps:** 125 mg, 250 mg, 500 mg **Oral Susp:** 62.5 mg/5 mL, 200 mL - $ Adult 10-14 days - $	**Children ≤40 kg:** 25-50 mg/kg/day (max 2 g/day) in divided doses every 6 hours for 10 days. **62.5 mg/5 mL @ 25 mg/kg/day** (double for 50 mg) 10 kg (22 lb) = 1 tsp (5 mL) Q6H 15 kg (33 lb) = 1½ tsp (7.5 mL) Q6H 20 kg (44 lb) = 2 tsp (10 mL) Q6H 40 kg (88 lb) = Use adult dose. **Children ≥40 kg and Adult:** 250-500 mg PO four times daily for 10 days.	**Food:** Take 1 hour before or 2 hours after meals. **Important side effects:** Bad taste, GI upset.
Erythromycin estolate or base* An alternative for patients with beta-lactam intolerance. (E-mycin®, Ilosone®) Generics available Pregnancy: B; Lactation: Unsafe **Estolate:** **Tabs:** 500 mg **Caps:** 250 mg **Oral Susp:** 125 mg/5 mL, 250 mg/5 mL 250 mg/5 mL Q12H × 10 days - $ **Base:** **Tabs:** 250 mg, 333 mg, 500 mg **Caps:** 250 mg 500 mg PO Q6H × 10 days - $	**Children:** 30-50 mg/kg/day (max 2 g/day) in two to four divided doses daily for 10 days. **125 mg/5 mL @ 30 mg/kg/day** 4 kg (10 lb) = ½ tsp (2.5 mL) Q12H 5-8 kg (11-18 lb) = 1 tsp (5 mL) Q12H 9-12 kg (20-26 lb) = 1 tsp (5 mL) Q8H 13-16 kg (29-35 lb) = 1 tsp (5 mL) Q6H or 2 tsp (10 mL) Q12H **250 mg/5 mL @ 30 mg/kg/day** 13-16 kg (29-35 lb) = 1 tsp (5 mL) Q12H 17-25 kg (37-55 lb) = 1½ tsp (7.5 mL) Q12H or 1 tsp (5 mL) Q8H 26-33 kg (57-72 lb) = 250 mg Q6H or 500 mg Q12H 30-50 kg (66-110 lb) = 500 mg Q8H **Adult:** Erythromycin base or estolate 500 mg PO four times daily for 10 days.	**Food:** May take with or without meals. Take with food if causes GI upset. **Important side effects:** GI upset, hepatitis.

(continued)

Drug, Its Forms and Dosage Increments	Children and Adult Dosages and Instructions	Information and Important Side Effects
SKIN – Impetigo Bullous (*Staphylococcus aureus*)		
Amoxicillin/clavulanate (Augmentin®) Pregnancy: B; Lactation: Unk **Q12H Formulations:** **Tabs:** 500 mg/125 mg, 875 mg/125 mg **Chewable Tabs:** 200 mg/28.5 mg, 400 mg/57 mg **Oral Susp:** 200 mg/28.5 mg/5 mL, 400 mg/57 mg/5 mL Child - $$$ Adult - >$$$$	**Children:** 40-45 mg amoxicillin component/kg/day (max 1600 mg/day) in divided doses two or three times daily for 10 days. **Q12H using 200 mg/5 mL susp @ 45 mg/kg/day** 9 kg (20 lb) = 1 tsp (or tab) (5 mL) Q12H 13 kg (29 lb) = 1½ tsp (or tab) (7.5 mL) Q12H 18 kg (40 lb) = 2 tsp (or tabs) (10 mL) Q12H **Q12H using 400 mg/5 mL susp @ 45 mg/kg/day** 18 kg (40 lb) = 1 tsp (or tab) (5 mL) Q12H 27 kg (59 lb) = 1½ tsp (or tab) (7.5 mL) Q12H 35 kg (77 lb) = 2 tsp (or tabs) (10 mL) Q12H >40 kg = Use adult dose (max 875 mg Q12H). **Adult:** 500-875 mg twice daily for 10 days. Note: Q12H dosing may improve compliance compared to Q8H dosing.	**Food:** Take with food to reduce diarrhea. **Important side effects:** Diarrhea (common), nausea, rash. **Use with caution in hepatic disease.** **Reduce dose in renal disease (CrCl <30 mL/min).**

Azithromycin* (Zithromax®) Pregnancy: B; Lactation: Unk **Tabs:** 250 mg and Z-Pak (500 mg × 1 day, then 250 mg daily × 4) **Oral Susp:** 100 mg/5 mL, 200 mg/5 mL 20-kg child - $$ Z-Pak - $$$	**Children ≥6 months:** 10 mg/kg/day (max 500 mg) once daily × 1 day, then 5 mg/kg/day (max 250 mg) once daily × 4 days **100 mg/5 mL** 10 kg (22 lb) = 1 tsp (5 mL)/day × 1 day, then ½ tsp (2.5 mL) daily for days 2-5. **200 mg/5 mL** 20 kg (44 lb) = 1 tsp (5 mL)/day × 1 day, then ½ tsp (2.5 mL) daily for days 2-5. 30 kg (66 lb) = 1.5 tsp/day × 1 day, then ¾ tsp daily for days 2-5. **Adult:** Dispense one Z-Pak.	**Food:** Oral suspension should be taken 1 hour before or 2 hours after food. Tablets may be taken without regard to food. **Important side effects:** Nausea, diarrhea, elevated LFTs.
Cephalexin (Keflex®) Generics available Pregnancy: B; Lactation: Unk	**Children:** 25-50 mg/kg/day (max 4 g/day) in divided doses two to four times daily for 10 days.	**Food:** May take with food if GI upset occurs. **Important side effects:** GI upset, diarrhea.
Clarithromycin* (Biaxin®, Biaxin XL®) Pregnancy: C; Lactation: Unk **Tabs:** 250 mg, 500 mg **Extended Release Tab (XL):** 500 mg **Oral Susp:** 125 mg/5 mL, 250 mg/5 mL 250 mg/5 mL Q12H × 10 days - $$$ 500 mg PO Q12H × 10 days - $$$$	**Children ≥6 months:** 15 mg/kg/day (max 1 g/day) in divided doses twice daily for 10 days. **125 mg/5 mL** 9 kg (20 lb) = ½ tsp (2.5 mL) Q12H 17 kg (37 lb) 1 tsp (5 mL) Q12H **250 mg/5 mL** 25 kg (55 lb) = ¾ tsp Q12H 33 kg (73 lb) = 1 tsp (5 mL) Q12H **Adult:** 250 mg PO twice daily for 10 days.	**Food:** Extended release tablet with food. Others without regard to food. **Important side effects:** Nausea, drug interactions. **Reduce dose in renal disease (CrCl <30 mL/min).**

(continued)

Drug, Its Forms and Dosage Increments	Children and Adult Dosages and Instructions	Information and Important Side Effects
Tabs: 250 mg, 500 mg, 1 g **Caps:** 250 mg, 500 mg **Oral Susp:** 125 mg/5 mL, 250 mg/5 mL 250 mg/5 mL Q6H × 10 days - <$ 500 mg PO Q6H × 10 days - $	**125 mg/5 mL @ 25 mg/kg/day** (double for 50 mg/kg) 10 kg (22 lb) = ½ tsp (2.5 mL) Q6H 15 kg (33 lb) = ¾ tsp Q6H 20 kg (44 lb) = 1 tsp (5 mL) Q6H **250 mg/5 mL @ 25 mg/kg/day** (double for 50 mg/kg) 20 kg (44 lb) = ½ tsp (2.5 mL) Q6H 40 kg (88 lb) = 1 tsp (5 mL) Q6H >40 kg = Use adult dose. **Adult:** 500 mg PO four times daily for 10 days.	**Reduce dose in renal disease (CrCl <40 mL/min).**
Dicloxacillin (Dynapen®) Generics available Pregnancy: B; Lactation: Unk **Caps:** 125 mg, 250 mg, 500 mg **Oral Susp:** 62.5 mg/5 mL, 200 mL $ Adult 10-14 days - $	**Children ≤40 kg:** 25-50 mg/kg/day (max 2 g/day) in divided doses every 6 hours for 10 days. **62.5 mg/5 mL @ 25 mg/kg/day** (double for 50 mg) 10 kg (22 lb) = 1 tsp (5 mL) Q6H 15 kg (33 lb) = 1½ tsp (7.5 mL) Q6H 20 kg (44 lb) = 2 tsp (10 mL) Q6H 40 kg (88 lb) = Use adult dose. **Children ≥40 kg and Adult:** 500 mg PO four times daily for 10 days.	**Food:** Take 1 hour before or 2 hours after meals. **Important side effects:** Bad taste, GI upset.

Erythromycin estolate or base*
Alternative for persons with beta-lactam intolerance.
(E-mycin®, Ilosone®)
Generics available
Pregnancy: B; Lactation: Unsafe
Estolate:
Tabs: 500 mg
Caps: 250 mg
Oral Susp: 125 mg/5 mL, 250 mg/5 mL
250 mg/5 mL Q12H × 10 days - $
Base:
Tabs: 250 mg, 333 mg, 500 mg
Caps: 250 mg
500 mg PO Q6H × 10 days - $

Children: 30-50 mg/kg/day estolate (max 2 g/day) PO in two to four divided doses daily for 10 days.
125 mg/5 mL @ 30 mg/kg/day
4 kg (10 lb) = ½ tsp (2.5 mL) Q12H
5-8 kg (11-18 lb) = 1 tsp (5 mL) Q12H
9-12 kg (20-26 lb) = 1 tsp (5 mL) Q8H
13-16 kg (29-35 lb) = 1 tsp (5 mL) Q6H or 2 tsp (10 mL) Q12H
250 mg/5 mL @ 30 mg/kg/day
13-16 kg (29-35 lb) = 1 tsp (5 mL) Q12H
17-25 kg (37-55 lb) = 1½ tsp (7.5 mL) Q12H or 1 tsp (5 mL) Q8H
26-33 kg (57-72 lb) = 250 mg Q6H or 500 mg Q12H
30-50 kg (66-110 lb) = 500 mg Q8H
Adult: Erythromycin base or estolate 500 mg PO four times daily for 10 days.

Food: May take with or without meals. Take with food if causes GI upset.
Important side effects: GI upset, hepatitis.

SKIN – Lice – Body (*Pediculus humanus corporis*)

General statement: Body lice does not usually require Rx therapy. Lice and nits reside within clothing. Discard clothing or wash in hot cycle and iron seams to eradicate infestation.

(continued)

Drug, Its Forms and Dosage Increments	Children and Adult Dosages and Instructions	Information and Important Side Effects
SKIN – Lice – Pubic (*Phthirus pubis*) May infest pubic area, axilla, coarse truncal hair, or eyelashes. **General statement:** Do not apply pediculicides to eyelids; use petrolatum to eyelid margins Q12H × 8 days, if needed. Symptomatic treatment may include oral antihistamines or topical corticosteroids to reduce pruritus. Secondary bacterial infections (often caused by scratching) may require antistaphylococcal therapy, such as dicloxacillin or cephalexin.		
Permethrin Nix Cream Rinse® Pregnancy: B; Lactation: Unk **Cream 5%:** For scabies only. **Cream Rinse 1%:** 60 mL 60-mL bottle (OTC) - $	**Children ≥2 months and Adult:** **Cream Rinse:** Wash hair and adjacent area, towel dry, saturate hair with Nix, and rinse after 10 minutes. Remove remaining nits with nit comb. One treatment eliminates infestations. Repeat only if live lice are seen after 7 days. Wash bedding and all clothing. Vacuum furniture and dispose of bag. Avoid contact with eye(s) and mucous membranes.	**Important side effects:** Mild temporary itching or erythema. **Caution:** Contraindicated if allergic to chrysanthemum flower.
Pyrethrins/piperonyl butoxide (RID®, A-200®, Pronto®, others) Pregnancy: C; Lactation: Unk 60-, 120-, 240-mL bottles (OTC) (120 mL adequate for two applications.) 120 mL - $	**Children and Adult:** Apply to dry hair. After 10 minutes, wash hair, rinse thoroughly. Comb out hair with nit comb. Repeat in 7-10 days. Wash bedding and all clothing. Vacuum furniture and dispose of bag.	**Important side effects:** Burning and pruritus. **Caution:** Contraindicated if allergic to ragweed or chrysanthemum flower.
SKIN – Lyme Disease, Acute Mild to Moderate (*Borrelia burgdorferi*)		
Amoxicillin (Amoxil®) Generics available	**Children:** 40-50 mg/kg/day (max 1500 mg/day) in divided doses three times daily for 21 days.	**Food:** May take with or without meals. **Important side effects:** Diarrhea and

Pregnancy: B; Lactation: Unsafe **Caps:** 250 mg, 500 mg - <$ **Tabs:** 500 mg, 875 mg - <$ **Chewable Tab:** 125 mg, 250 mg, **Susp:** 125 mg/5 mL, 250 mg/5 mL, - $ **Oral drops:** 50 mg/mL	**250 mg/tsp @ 40 mg/kg/day** 10 kg (22 lb) = 3 mL Q8H 15 kg (33 lb) = 1 tsp (5 mL) Q8H 20 kg (44 lb) = 1½ tsp (7.5 mL) Q8H ≥ 30 kg (66 lb) = Use adult dose. **Adult:** 500 mg PO three times daily for 21 days.	nausea. May cause nonallergic maculopapular rash. **Reduce dose in renal disease (CrCl <30 mL/min).**
Doxycycline* (Vibramycin®) Generics available Pregnancy: D; Lactation: Unsafe **Caps:** 50 mg, 100 mg - <$ **Tabs:** 50 mg, 100 mg - <$ **Oral Susp:** 25 mg/5 mL - $ **Syrup:** 50 mg/5 mL - $$	**Children:** 2-4 mg/kg/day (max 200 mg/day) in 2 divided doses for 21 days. **Children ≥8 years and Adult:** 100 mg PO twice daily for 21 days. A drug of choice, especially for persons intolerant to beta-lactams. Consider in younger children if true beta-lactam allergy. Especially useful if coinfection with ehrlichiosis suspected.	**Food:** May take with food if GI upset occurs. Take 1 hour before or 2 hours after antacids, iron, milk, or other dairy products. Take with full glass of water to prevent esophagitis. **Important side effects:** Photosensitivity, (use sunscreen), esophagitis. May discolor fingernails. Low chance of staining teeth in young children, avoid repeated courses.
Cefuroxime axetil (Ceftin®) Pregnancy: B; Lactation: Unsafe **Tabs:** 125 mg, 250 mg, 500 mg **Oral Susp:** 125 mg/5 mL, 250 mg/5 mL 125 mg/5 mL Q12H × 10 days - $$ 250 mg PO Q12H × 10 days - $$$$	**Children >3 months to 12 years:** 30 mg/kg/day (max 1 g/day) in divided doses twice daily for 21 days. **125 mg/5 mL @ 30 mg/kg/day** 8 kg (18 lb) = 1 tsp (5 mL) Q12H 12.5 kg (27 lb) = 1½ tsp (7.5 mL) Q12H 17 kg (37 lb) = 2 tsp (10 mL) Q12H 25 kg (55 lb) = 3tsp (15 mL) Q12H >33 kg (73 lb) = Use adult dose. **Children ≥13 years or Adult:** 500 mg PO twice daily for 21 days.	**Food:** Take suspension with food. Tablets may be taken without regard to food. **Reduce dose in renal disease (CrCl <30 mL/min).**

(continued)

Drug, Its Forms and Dosage Increments	Children and Adult Dosages and Instructions	Information and Important Side Effects
Erythromycin estolate or base* (E-mycin®, Ilosone®) Generics available Pregnancy: B; Lactation: Unsafe **Note:** Higher rate of clinical failure compared to amoxicillin and doxycycline. Use only for patients with documented allergy to beta-lactams and tetracyclines. **Estolate:** **Tabs:** 500 mg **Caps:** 250 mg **Oral Susp:** 125 mg/5 mL, 250 mg/5 mL 250 mg/5 mL Q12H × 10 days $ **Base:** **Tabs:** 250 mg, 333 mg, 500 mg **Caps:** 250 mg 500 mg PO Q6H × 10 days - $	**Children:** 30-40 mg/kg/day estolate (max 2 g/day) in two to four divided doses daily for 21 days. **125 mg/5 mL @ 30 mg/kg/day** 4 kg (10 lb) = ½ tsp (2.5 mL) Q12H 5-8 kg (11-18 lb) = 1 tsp (5 mL) Q12H 9-12 kg (20-26 lb) = 1 tsp (5 mL) Q8H 13-16 kg (29-35 lb) = 1 tsp (5 mL) Q6H **250 mg/5 mL @ 30 mg/kg/day** 13-16 kg (29-35 lb) = 1 tsp (5 mL) Q12H 17-25 kg (37-55 lb) = 1 tsp (5 mL) Q8H 26-33 kg (57-72 lb) = 250 mg Q6H **Adult:** Erythromycin base or estolate 250 mg PO four times daily for 21 days.	**Food:** May take with or without meals. Take with food if causes GI upset. **Important side effects:** GI upset, hepatitis.
Penicillin V Potassium (Pen Vee K®) Generics available Pregnancy: B; Lactation: Unsafe **Tabs:** 125 mg, 250 mg, 500 mg - <$	**Children:** Inadequate information to recommend use in children at this time. **Adult:** 500 mg PO every 6 hours for 21 days.	**Food:** Take 1 hour before or 2 hours after meals. May take with food if GI upset occurs. **Important side effects:** Nausea, rash. Use cautiously if history of seizures.

SKIN – Lyme Disease, Acute Infection, Pregnant Woman (*Borrelia burgdorferi*)

Drug	Dosage	Notes
Amoxicillin (Amoxil®) Generics available Pregnancy: B; Lactation: Unsafe **Caps:** 250 mg, 500 mg - $ **Tabs:** 500 mg - $	**Adult:** 500 mg PO three times daily for 21 days.	**Food:** May take with or without meals. **Important side effects:** Diarrhea and nausea. May cause nonallergic maculopapular rash. **Reduce dose in renal disease (CrCl <30 mL/min).**

SKIN – Lyme Disease – Arthritis or Isolated Facial Nerve Palsy (*Borrelia burgdorferi*)

Drug	Dosage	Notes
Amoxicillin (Amoxil®) Generics available Pregnancy: B; Lactation: Unsafe **Caps:** 250 mg, 500 mg - <$ **Tabs:** 500 mg, 875 mg - <$ **Chewable Tab:** 125 mg, 200 mg, 250 mg, 400 mg - <$ **Susp:** 125 mg/5 mL, 250 mg/5 mL, 400 mg/5 mL - <$ **Oral drops:** 50 mg/mL	**Children:** **Facial Paralysis:** 40-50 mg/kg/day (max 1500 mg/day) in divided doses three times daily for 21-30 days. **Arthritis:** Four times daily for 28 days. **250 mg/tsp @ 40 mg/kg/day** 10 kg (22 lb) = ½ tsp (2.5 mL) Q8H 15 kg (33 lb) = ¾ tsp Q8H 20 kg (44 lb) = 1 tsp (5 mL) Q8H >20 kg = Use adult dose. **Adult:** **Facial paralysis:** 500 mg PO three times daily for 21-30 days. **Arthritis:** Four times daily for 28 days	**Food:** May take with or without meals. **Important side effects:** Diarrhea and nausea. May cause nonallergic maculopapular rash.
Doxycycline* (Vibramycin®) Generics available Pregnancy: D; Lactation: Unsafe	**Children:** 2-4 mg/kg/day (max 200 mg/day) in two divided doses for 21-30 days (facial paralysis) or 28 days (arthritis). (Ped Infect Dis J 1990;18:913-925.)	**Food:** May take with food if GI upset occurs. Take 1 hour before or 2 hours after antacids, iron, milk, or other dairy

(continued)

Drug, Its Forms and Dosage Increments	Children and Adult Dosages and Instructions	Information and Important Side Effects
Note: A drug of choice, especially for persons intolerant to beta-lactams. Consider in younger children if true beta-lactam allergy. **Caps:** 50 mg, 100 mg - <$ **Tabs:** 100 mg - <$ **Oral Susp:** 25 mg/5 mL - <$ **Syrup:** 50 mg/5 mL	**Children ≥8 years and Adult:** 100 mg PO twice daily for 21-30 days (facial paralysis) or 28 days (arthritis).	products. Take with full glass of water to prevent esophagitis. **Important side effects:** Photosensitivity, (use sunscreen), esophagitis. May discolor fingernails. Low chance of staining teeth in young children; avoid repeated courses.
Ceftriaxone* (Rocephin®) Pregnancy: B; Lactation: Unk	**Children:** 100 mg/kg/day (up to 2 g) IV once daily for 14-28 days. **Adult:** 2 g IV once daily for 14-28 days.	**Important side effects:** Pain with injection.

SKIN – Mastitis (*Staphylococcus aureus*) See cellulitis for more therapy options.

Drug, Its Forms and Dosage Increments	Children and Adult Dosages and Instructions	Information and Important Side Effects
Cephalexin (Keflex®) Generics available Pregnancy: B; Lactation: Unk **Tabs:** 250 mg, 500 mg, 1 g **Caps:** 250 mg, 500 mg **Oral Susp:** 125 mg/5 mL, 250 mg/5 mL 250 mg/5 mL Q6H × 10 days - <$ 500 mg PO Q6H × 10 days - $	**Adult:** 500 mg PO four times daily for 10-14 days.	**Food:** May take with food if GI upset occurs. **Important side effects:** GI upset, diarrhea. **Reduce dose in renal disease (CrCl <40 mL/min).**

Clindamycin* (Cleocin®) Generics available Pregnancy: B; Lactation: Unk **Caps:** 75 mg, 150 mg, 300 mg 300 mg PO Q6H × 14 days - $$$	**Adult:** 300 mg PO four times daily for 10-14 days. ***May cause severe colitis.** Encourage patient to report severe, persistent, or bloody diarrhea.	**Food:** May take with or without meals. Take with full glass of water to prevent esophagitis. **Important side effects:** Diarrhea, may be severe. Nausea and esophagitis.
Dicloxacillin (Dynapen®) Generics available Pregnancy: B; Lactation: Unk **Caps:** 250 mg, 500 mg 10-14 days - $	**Adult:** 500 mg PO four times daily for 10-14 days.	**Food:** Take 1 hour before or 2 hours after meals. **Important side effects:** Bad taste, GI upset.

SKIN – Onychomycosis Toenails, Fingernails (*Tinea unguium*) Long-term efficacy of terbinafine may be superior to itraconazole.

Fluconazole* Diflucan® Pregnancy: C; Lactation: Unsafe **Tabs:** 50 mg, 100 mg, 150 mg, 200 mg - >$$$$	**Fingernail** **Children: N/A** **Adult:** 150-300 mg once per week for 3-6 months. **Toenail** **Children: N/A** **Adult:** 150-300 mg once per week for 6-12 months.	**Food:** May take with or without meals. **Important side effects:** Nausea, vomiting, diarrhea, dizziness. Advise patient to report any prodromal signs of liver failure. Drug interactions may be significant. Consult a pharmacist.
Itraconazole* (Sporanox®) Pregnancy: C; Lactation: Unsafe	**Fingernails** **Children:** Not approved. **Adult:** 200 mg PO once daily for 6-12 weeks	**Food:** Avoid grapefruit products while taking. Take capsules with food. Take oral solution on an empty stomach. Not

(continued)

Drug, Its Forms and Dosage Increments	Children and Adult Dosages and Instructions	Information and Important Side Effects
Caps: 100 mg - >$$$$	OR **Pulse dosing:** 200 mg twice daily one week then off for three weeks. Repeat two times for fingernails. **Toenails** **Children:** Not approved. **Adult:** 200 mg PO once daily for 3 months OR **Pulse dosing:** 200 mg twice daily one week then off for 3 weeks. Repeat three to four times for toenails.	well absorbed with acid-suppressing drugs. **Important side effects:** Advise patient to report any prodromal signs of liver failure. **Caution:** May cause hepatitis. Use with caution in persons with history of liver disease. Consider periodic liver function tests. May cause or contribute to congestive heart failure or cardiac dysrhythmias. Use with caution in persons with history of cardiac disease. Use for onychomycosis is contraindicated in patients with history of ventricular dysfunction or CHF. Use is contraindicated in any patient taking cisapride, dofetilide, quinidine, midazolam, triazolam, pimozide, lovastatin, or simvastatin. Not well absorbed with acid-suppressing drug. Has caused bone defects and changes in tooth appearance in rats; implications for humans are not established.

Terbinafine*
(Lamisil®)
Pregnancy: B; Lactation: Unsafe
Tabs: 250 mg - >$$$$

Fingernails
Children (>2 years) <20 kg: 62.5 mg Q24H for 6 weeks.
20-40 kg: 125 mg Q24H for 6 weeks.
≥40 kg and Adult: 250 mg Q24H for 6 weeks.
Toenails
Children (>2 years) <20 kg: 62.5 mg Q24H for 12 weeks.
20-40 kg: 125 mg Q24H for 12 weeks.
≥40 kg and Adult: 250 mg PO once daily for 12 weeks.

Food: May take with or without meals.
Important side effects: Ocular changes, rash, neutropenia, hepatobiliary dysfunction, nausea. Advise patient to report any prodromal signs of liver failure. Liver failure and death have occurred.
Baseline LFTs should be obtained and patient should be advised to contact provider if any side effects occur.

SKIN – Paronychia (*Staphylococcus aureus*) In thumbsuckers and nailbiters may also be caused by Group A *Streptococcus* or anaerobes. May require incision & drainage.

Dicloxacillin
(Dynapen®)
Generics available
Pregnancy: B; Lactation: Unk
Caps: 125 mg, 250 mg, 500 mg
Oral Susp: 62.5 mg/5 mL, 200 mL - $
Adult 10-14 days - $

Children ≤40 kg: 25-50 mg/kg/day (max 2 g/day) in divided doses every 6 hours for 10-14 days.
62.5 mg/5 mL @ 25 mg/kg/day (double for 50 mg/kg)
10 kg (22 lb) = 1 tsp (5 mL) Q6H
15 kg (33 lb) = 1½ tsp (7.5 mL) Q6H
20 kg (44 lb) = 2 tsp (10 mL) Q6H
40 kg (88 lb) = Use adult dose.
Children ≥40 kg and Adult: 250-500 mg PO four times daily for 10-14 days.

Food: Take 1 hour before or 2 hours after meals.
Important side effects: Bad taste, GI upset.

(continued)

Drug, Its Forms and Dosage Increments	Children and Adult Dosages and Instructions	Information and Important Side Effects
Cephalexin (Keflex®) Generics available Pregnancy: B; Lactation: Unk **Tabs:** 250 mg, 500 mg, 1 g **Caps:** 250 mg, 500 mg **Oral Susp:** 125 mg/5 mL, 250 mg/5 mL 250 mg/5 mL Q6H × 10 days - <$ 500 mg PO Q6H × 10 days - $	**Children:** 25-50 mg/kg/day (max 4 g/day) in divided doses two to four times daily for 10-14 days. **125 mg/5 mL @ 25 mg/kg/day** (double for 50 mg/kg) 10 kg (22 lb) = ½ tsp (2.5 mL) Q6H 15 kg (33 lb) = ¾ tsp Q6H 20 kg (44 lb) = 1 tsp (5 mL) Q6H **250 mg/5 mL @ 25 mg/kg/day** (double for 50 mg/kg) 20 kg (44 lb) = ½ tsp (2.5 mL) Q6H 40 kg (88 lb) = 1 tsp (5 mL) Q6H >40 kg = Use adult dose. **Adult:** 250-500 mg four times daily for 10-14 days.	**Food:** May take with food if GI upset occurs. **Important side effects:** GI upset, diarrhea. **Reduce dose in renal disease (CrCl <40 mL/min).**
Amoxicillin/clavulanate (Augmentin®) DOC for thumbsuckers and nailbiters. Pregnancy: B; Lactation: Unk **Q12H Formulations:** **Tabs:** 500 mg/125 mg, 875 mg/125 mg **Chewable Tabs:** 200 mg/28.5 mg, 400 mg/57 mg	**Children:** 40-45 mg amoxicillin component/kg/day (max 1600 mg/day) in divided doses two or three times daily for 10-14 days. **Q12H using 200 mg/5 mL susp @ 45 mg/kg/day** 9 kg (20 lb) = 1 tsp (5 mL) Q12H 13 kg (29 lb) = 1½ tsp (7.5 mL) Q12H 18 kg (40 lb) = 2 tsp (10 mL) Q12H	**Food:** Take with food to reduce diarrhea. **Important side effects:** Diarrhea (common), nausea, rash. **Use with caution in hepatic disease.** **Reduce dose in renal disease (CrCl <30 mL/min).**

Drug	Dosage	Notes
Oral Susp: 200 mg/28.5 mg/5 mL, 400 mg/57 mg/5 mL Child - $$$ Adult - >$$$$	**Q12H using 400 mg/5 mL susp @ 45 mg/kg/day** 18 kg (40 lb) = 1 tsp (5 mL) Q12H 27 kg (59 lb) = 1½ tsp (7.5 mL) Q12H 35 kg (77 lb) = 2 tsp (10 mL) Q12H >40 kg = Use adult dose (max 875 mg Q12H). **Adult:** 500-875 mg twice daily for 10-14 days.	
Clindamycin* (Cleocin®) Generics available Pregnancy: B; Lactation: Unk **Caps:** 75 mg, 150 mg, 300 mg **Oral Solution:** 75 mg/5 mL 150 mg/10 mL Q8H × 10 days - $$$ 300 mg PO Q6H × 10 days - $$	**Children:** 10-15 mg/kg/day (max 1.8 g/day) in divided doses PO three or four 10-14 days. **10 mg/kg/day divided Q8H @ 75 mg/5 mL** 10 kg (22 lb) = ½ tsp (2.5 mL) Q8H 20 kg (44 lb) = 1 tsp (5 mL) Q8H 30 kg (66 lb) = 1½ tsp (7.5 mL) Q8H 40 kg (88 lb) = 2 tsp (10 mL) Q8H >40 kg = Use adult dose. **Adult:** 150-300 mg PO four times daily for 10-14 days.	**Food:** May take with or without meals. Take with full glass of water to prevent esophagitis. **Important side effects:** Diarrhea, may be severe. Nausea and esophagitis. ***May cause severe colitis.** Encourage patient to report severe, persistent, or bloody diarrhea.

SKIN – Tinea Corporis, Tinea Cruris, Tinea Pedis – Topical Treatment (*Trichophyton sp.*)

Drug	Dosage	Notes
Clotrimazole (OTC)* (Lotrimin®, Mycelex®)	**Children and Adult:** Apply after washing and drying twice daily for 2-3 weeks, or for	**Avoid contact with eye(s).**

(continued)

Drug, Its Forms and Dosage Increments	Children and Adult Dosages and Instructions	Information and Important Side Effects
Generics available Pregnancy: B; Lactation: Unk **Cream 1%:** 30 g, 15 g **Lotion 1%:** 20 mL, 30 mL **Topical Solution 1%:** 10 mL, 30 mL	several days after all signs of infection have cleared.	
Econazole* (Spectazole®) Pregnancy: C; Lactation: Unk **Cream 1%** Available in 15, 30, and 85 g	**Children and Adult:** Apply after washing and drying daily for 2-4 weeks or until cleared.	**Avoid contact with eye(s).** Wash hands after application. Wear well ventilated shoes.
Miconazole (OTC)* (Monistat-Derm®, Micatin®, Ting®) Generics Available Pregnancy: C; Lactation: Unk **Cream 2%, Powder 2%** **Topical Solution 2%, Spray 2%**	**Children and Adult:** Apply after washing and drying twice daily for 2-3 weeks or for several days after all signs of infection have cleared.	**Avoid contact with eye(s).**
Terbinafine* (Lamisil®) Pregnancy: B; Lactation: Unsafe **Cream 1% (OTC):** 15 g, 30 g - $$ **Gel (Rx only) 1%:** 5 g, 15 g, 30 g	**Children:** Not recommended. **Adult (Cream):** Apply after washing and drying once or twice daily for at least one week, but do not exceed 4 weeks. **Adult (Gel):** Apply to affected area once daily for 7 days.	**Avoid contact with eye(s), nose, lips. Notify prescriber if skin or eye(s) become yellow.**
Tolnaftate (OTC)* (Tinactin®, Ting®)	**Children and Adult:** Apply after washing and drying two or three times daily for 2-4	**Avoid contact with eye(s).**

Generics available Pregnancy: C; Lactation: Unknown **Spray Liquid, Powder 1%** **Cream 1%, Topical Gel, Liquid, or Powder 1%**	weeks, or for several days after all signs of infection have cleared.	

SKIN – Tinea Corporis, Tinea Cruris, Tinea Pedis – Oral Treatment (*Trichophyton sp.*)

<u>Griseofulvin microsize</u> (Grifulvin-V®, Fulvicin U/F®) Generics available Pregnancy: C; Lactation: Unk **Tabs:** 250 mg, 500 mg **Caps:** 250 mg **Oral Susp:** 125 mg/5 mL (120 mL = $$) Adult 4-6 weeks - $$-$$$	**Children >2 years:** 10-20 mg/kg/day (max 500 mg) **Using 125 mg/5 mL @ 10 mg/kg/day** 5 kg (11 lb) = 2 mL Q24H 7.5 kg (16 lb) = 3 mL Q24H 10 kg (22 lb) = 4 mL Q24H 12.5 kg (28 lb) = 5 mL (1 tsp) Q24H 15 kg (33 lb) = 6 mL Q24H 20 kg (44 lb) = 8 mL Q24H 25 kg (55 lb) = 10 mL (2 tsp) Q24H or 250 mg tab/cap Q24H **Adult:** 500 mg once daily. **Duration:** Tinea corporis 2-4 weeks Tinea pedis 4-8 weeks	**Food:** Food decreases stomach upset. Fatty meals increase absorption. **Important side effects:** Rash, urticaria, headache, dizziness. **Caution:** In patients with liver problems and systemic lupus, avoid prolonged exposure to sunlight. Avoid alcohol.
Fluconazole* (Diflucan®) Pregnancy: C; Lactation: Unsafe **Tabs:** 50 mg, 100 mg, 150 mg - $$-$$$	**Children: N/A** **Adult:** 150 mg once per week for 2-4 weeks.	**Food:** May take with or without meals. **Important side effects:** Nausea, vomiting, diarrhea, dizziness. Advise patient to report any prodromal signs of

(continued)

Drug, Its Forms and Dosage Increments	Children and Adult Dosages and Instructions	Information and Important Side Effects
		liver failure. Potentially significant drug interactions. Consult a pharmacist.
Itraconazole* (Sporanox®) Pregnancy: C; Lactation: Unsafe **Caps:** 100 mg - >$$$$	**Children:** Not approved. **Adult**: 100 mg daily for 2 weeks or 200 mg once daily for 7 days.	**Food:** Avoid grapefruit products while taking. Take capsules with food. Take oral solution on an empty stomach. Not well absorbed with acid-suppressing drugs. **Important side effects:** Advise patient to report any prodromal signs of liver failure. Potentially significant drug interactions. Consult a pharmacist. **Caution:** May cause hepatitis. Use with caution in persons with history of liver disease. Consider periodic liver function tests. May cause or contribute to congestive heart failure or cardiac dysrhythmias. Use with caution in persons with history of cardiac disease. Use for onychomycosis is contraindicated in patients with history of ventricular dysfunction or CHF. Use is contraindicated in any patient taking cisapride, dofetilide, quinidine, midazolam, triazolam, pimozide, lovastatin, or simvastatin. Not well

Drug	Dosage	Comments
		absorbed with acid-suppressing drug. Has caused bone defects and changes in tooth appearance in rats; implications for humans are not established.
Terbinafine* (Lamisil®) Pregnancy: B; Lactation: Unsafe **Tabs:** 250 mg - >$$$$	**Adult:** 250 mg PO once daily for 14 days. Baseline LFTs should be obtained, and patient should be advised to contact provider if any side effects occur.	**Food:** May take with or without meals. **Important side effects:** Ocular changes, rash, neutropenia, hepatobiliary dysfunction, nausea. Advise patient to report any prodromal signs of liver failure.

SKIN – Tinea Versicolor – Topical Treatment (*Malassezia furfur, Pityrosporum orbiculare*) **General statement:** Creams may be practical for small areas but are expensive and difficult to apply to extensive infection. Shampoo and lotion are easy to apply. Oral therapy for extensive infection, frequent recurrence, or infection resistant to topical therapy. Recurrences are common. Once-a-month shampoo or lotion may reduce recurrences.

Drug	Dosage	Comments
Clotrimazole (OTC) (Lotrimin®, Mycelex®) Generics available Pregnancy: B; Lactation: Unk **Cream 1%:** 30 g	**Children and Adult:** Apply twice daily for 2-4 weeks.	Avoid contact with eye(s).
Ketoconazole Shampoo (Nizoral®) Pregnancy: C; Lactation: Unsafe **Shampoo 2%:** 120 mL **Cream 2%:** 15 g, 30 g, 60 g	**Children and Adult:** Apply to dampened skin. Leave on 5 minutes, then rinse. Repeat daily for 1-3 days. **Cream:** Apply once daily for 2 weeks.	**Caution:** Avoid contact with eye(s) and mucous membranes. May remove curl from permanently waved hair.

(continued)

Drug, Its Forms and Dosage Increments	Children and Adult Dosages and Instructions	Information and Important Side Effects
Econazole (Spectazole®) Pregnancy: C; Lactation: Unk **Cream:** 15 g, 30 g, 85 g	**Children and Adult:** Apply once daily for 2-4 weeks.	Avoid contact with eye(s). Wash Hands after application.
Miconazole (Monistat-Derm®) Pregnancy: C; Lactation: Unk **Cream 2%:** 15 g, 30 g	**Children and Adult:** Apply twice daily for 2-4 weeks.	Avoid contact with eye(s).
Selenium sulfide 2.5%* (Selsun®, Excel®) Generics available Pregnancy: C; Lactation: Unk **Shampoo 1%:** Selsun Blue® 1% (OTC) **Shampoo and Lotion 2.5%** 240-mL bottle - $3.25	**Children and Adult:** Apply 2.5% lotion or shampoo to affected areas and lather with a small amount of water. Keep on skin for 10 minutes, then rinse thoroughly. Repeat once daily for 7-14 days or alternatively apply overnight once per week for 2 weeks.	Wash hands after treatment, avoid contact with eye(s). **Important side effects:** May irritate skin and discolor hair or jewelry. Rinse thoroughly after use.

SKIN – Tinea Versicolor – Oral Treatment (*Malassezia furfur, Pityrosporum orbiculare*)

Drug, Its Forms and Dosage Increments	Children and Adult Dosages and Instructions	Information and Important Side Effects
Fluconazole* (Diflucan®) Pregnancy: C; Lactation: Unsafe **Tabs:** 50 mg, 100 mg, 150 mg, 200 mg - <$	**Children:** Not approved. **Adult:** 400 mg PO once. Repeat once a month if needed.	**Food:** May take with or without meals. **Important side effects:** Nausea, vomiting, diarrhea, dizziness. Potentially significant drug interactions. Consult a pharmacist.

Itraconazole* (Sporanox®) Pregnancy: C; Lactation: Unsafe **Caps:** 100 mg - $$	**Children:** Not approved. **Adult:** 200 mg once daily for 5-7 days.	**Food:** Avoid grapefruit products while taking. Take capsules with food. Take oral solution on an empty stomach. Not well absorbed with acid-suppressing drugs. **Caution:** May cause hepatitis. Use with caution in persons with history of liver disease. Consider periodic liver function tests. May cause or contribute to congestive heart failure or cardiac dysrhythmias. Use with caution in persons with history of cardiac disease. Use for onychomycosis is contraindicated in patients with history of ventricular dysfunction or CHF. Use is contraindicated in any patient taking cisapride, dofetilide, quinidine, midazolam, triazolam, pimozide, lovastatin, or simvastatin. Not well absorbed with acid-suppressing drug. Has caused bone defects and changes in tooth appearance in rats; implications for humans are not established.
Ketoconazole* (Nizoral®) Pregnancy: C; Lactation: Unsafe	**Children ≥2 years:** 3.3-6.6 mg/kg once daily (max 400 mg/day) once per week for 3 weeks.	**Food:** Food may increase absorption. Do not take with acid-suppressing agents.

(continued)

Drug, Its Forms and Dosage Increments	Children and Adult Dosages and Instructions	Information and Important Side Effects
Tabs: 200 mg - \$-\$\$	**200 mg @ 4-5 mg/kg daily** 25 lb (11 kg) = ¼ tab Q24H 50 lb (22 kg) = ½ tab Q24H 75 lb (33 kg) = ¾ tab Q24H 100 lb (45 kg) = 1 tab Q24H **Adult:** 400 mg as a single dose once per week for 3 weeks or 200 mg daily for 5-7 days.	**Important side effects:** Liver toxicity, nausea, dizziness, headache.

SKIN – Scabies (*Sarcoptes scabiei*) **General statement:** Itching may continue for several weeks following successful therapy and should not be viewed as failure. Oral antihistamines or topical corticosteroids may provide symptomatic relief. Clothing and bedding should be washed in hot water and dried in hot dryer. Treat close contacts if needed.

Drug, Its Forms and Dosage Increments	Children and Adult Dosages and Instructions	Information and Important Side Effects
Permethrin 5% **Preferred to lindane.** (Elimite®) Generics available Pregnancy: B; Lactation: Unk **Cream 5%:** 60 g	**Children ≥2 months and Adult:** Massage into all areas of skin from chin line to toe (head to toe in infants), leave on for 8-14 hours, then wash off thoroughly. May repeat in 1 week if live mites are seen.	**Important side effects:** Mild temporary itching, burning, or erythema. **Caution:** Avoid contact with eye(s) and mucous membranes. Contraindicated if allergic to chrysanthemum flower.
Lindane 1% (G-well®, Kwell®) Generics available Pregnancy: B; Lactation: Unk **Lotion 1%:** 30 ml, 60 mL (30-60 mL should be sufficient quantity for child ≥6 years to adult for one application).	**Children and Adult:** Apply a thin layer and massage well into skin from chin line to toes (head to toe in infants). Wash off after 6 hours (infant), 6-8 hours (child), or 8-12 hours (adult). Do not repeat sooner than 1 week and only if live mites are seen.	**Important side effects:** Nausea, vomiting, headache, seizure may be signs of excessive absorption. Contact healthcare provider immediately.

GASTROINTESTINAL – *H. pylori* Treatment (*Helicobacter pylori*) Numerous regimens are generally equally effective, but vary in tolerability, convenience, duration, and cost.

Regimen #1 (3 Drugs)		
Lansoprazole (Prevacid®) Pregnancy: B; Lactation: Unk	30 mg twice daily for 10 days.	**Food:** Take 15-30 minutes before AM and PM meals.
and		
Clarithromycin* (Biaxin®) Pregnancy: C; Lactation: Unk	500 mg twice daily for 10 days.	**Important side effects:** Drug interactions.
and		
Amoxicillin (Amoxil®) Generics available Pregnancy: B; Lactation: Unk	1,000 mg twice daily for 10 days.	**Food:** May take with or without meals. **Important side effects:** Diarrhea and nausea. May cause nonallergic maculopapular rash.
Regimen #2 (3 Drugs)		
Omeprazole (Prilosec®) Pregnancy: C; Lactation: Unk	20 mg twice daily for 10 days.	**Food:** Take 15-30 minutes before AM and PM meals.
and		
Clarithromycin* (Biaxin®) Pregnancy: C; Lactation: Unk	500 mg twice daily for 10 days.	**Important side effects:** Drug interactions.
and		
Amoxicillin (Amoxil®) Generics available Pregnancy: B; Lactation: Unk	1,000 mg twice daily for 10 days.	**Food:** May take with or without meals. **Important side effects:** Diarrhea and nausea. May cause nonallergic maculopapular rash.

(continued)

Drug, Its Forms and Dosage Increments	Children and Adult Dosages and Instructions	Information and Important Side Effects
Regimen #3 (4 Drugs)		
Omeprazole (Prilosec®) Pregnancy: C; Lactation: Unk **and**	20 mg PO twice daily for 10 days.	**Food:** Take 15-30 minutes before AM and PM meals.
Bismuth (Pepto-Bismol®) Pregnancy: C; (D third trimester) Lactation: Unknown **and**	2 × 262 mg tablets PO four times daily for 10 days.	**Important side effects:** May darken stools or tongue. **Drug interactions:** Salicylates, warfarin Avoid, or use with caution, in history of aspirin allergy, renal disease, GI bleed.
Tetracycline (Sumycin®) Generics available Pregnancy: D; Lactation: Unsafe **Caps:** 250 mg, 500 mg **Tabs:** 250 mg, 500 mg **and**	500 mg PO four times daily for 10 days.	**Food:** 1hour before or 2 hours after meals. Do not take with dairy products, antacids, calcium, zinc, or iron products. Take with large glass of water to prevent esophagitis. **Important side effects:** GI upset, esophagitis, photosensitivity, discoloration of fingernails.
Metronidazole* (Flagyl®) Generics available Pregnancy: B; Lactation: Unk **Tabs:** 250 mg, 500 mg	500 mg PO three times daily for 10 days.	**Food:** Administer on empty stomach unless GI upset occurs, then with food. **Important side effects:** Dizziness, headache, confusion, seizures, nausea, metallic taste, insomnia, paresthesias. **Caution:** May cause disulfiram-like reaction; avoid alcohol.

GASTROINTESTINAL – Diarrhea, Acute, Empiric Therapy (*Shigella*, *Escherichia coli*, *Salmonella*) **Note:** Most patients do not require antimicrobial therapy. Consider empiric therapy for patients with fever, bloody stools, or prolonged symptoms. Empiric antibiotic therapy for acute diarrhea in children is not recommended. Early antibiotic therapy, especially with TMP/SMX, in children infected with *E. coli* 0157:H7, may be associated with hemolytic uremic syndrome.

Ciprofloxacin* (Cipro®) Pregnancy: C; Lactation: Unsafe **Tabs:** 250 mg, 500 mg, 750 mg - $$-$$$$ Use with antimotility drug such as loperamide (Imodium®) if no fever or blood in stool.	**≥18 and Adult, Mild to Moderate:** Fluids +/– antimotility drugs. **≥18 and Adult, Severe:** 500 mg PO twice daily for 3-5 days.	**Food:** Take on empty stomach 1 hour before or 2 hours after a meal. May take with food if it causes GI upset, but avoid large amounts of dairy products. May take 2 hours before or 6 hours after sucralfate, antacids, aluminum, magnesium, calcium, zinc, iron, sucralfate, vitamins, or mineral supplements. **Important side effects:** Photosensitivity, dizziness. **Reduce dose in renal disease (CrCl <50 mL/min).**
Levofloxacin* (Levaquin®) Pregnancy: C; Lactation: Unsafe **Tabs:** 250 mg, 500 mg - $$ Use with antimotility drug such as loperamide (Imodium®) if no fever or blood in stool.	**≥18 and Adult:** 500 mg Q24H × 3-5 days.	**Food:** May take with or without meals. Do not take within 2 hours of antacids, magnesium, calcium supplements, aluminum, sucralfate, vitamins, or minerals (iron or zinc). **Important side effects:** Photosensitivity, dizziness. **Reduce dose in renal disease (CrCl <50 mL/min).**

(continued)

Drug, Its Forms and Dosage Increments	Children and Adult Dosages and Instructions	Information and Important Side Effects
Trimethoprim/Sulfamethoxazole* (Bactrim®, Septra®, Cotrim®) Generics available Pregnancy: C; Lactation: Unsafe **Single Strength (SS) Tabs:** 80 mg/400 mg - <$ **Double Strength (DS) Tabs:** 160 mg/800 mg - <$ **Susp:** 40 mg/200 mg/5 mL	**Adult, Mild to Moderate:** Fluids ± antimotility drugs. **Adult, Severe:** 1 DS Tab PO twice daily for 3-5 days.	**Food:** May take without regard to food. Encourage fluids. **Important side effects:** Photosensitivity, rash. **Reduce dose in renal disease (CrCl <30 mL/min).**

GASTROINTESTINAL – Diarrhea, Acute, Traveler's, Mild to Severe (*Shigella, E. coli, Salmonella*)

Drug, Its Forms and Dosage Increments	Children and Adult Dosages and Instructions	Information and Important Side Effects
Ciprofloxacin* (Cipro®) Pregnancy: C; Lactation: Unsafe **Tabs:** 250 mg, 500 mg, 750 mg - $$ Use with antimotility drug such as loperamide (Imodium®) if no fever or blood in stool.	**≥18 and Adult, Mild to Moderate:** 750 mg PO × 1 dose. **≥18 and Adult, Severe:** 500 mg twice daily × 3 days.	**Food:** Take on empty stomach 1 hour before or 2 hours after a meal. May take with food if it causes GI upset, but avoid large amounts of dairy products. May take 2 hours before or 6 hours after sucralfate, antacids, aluminum, magnesium, calcium, zinc, iron, sucralfate, vitamins, or mineral supplements. **Important side effects:** Photosensitivity, dizziness. **Reduce dose in renal disease (CrCl <50 mL/min).**

Levofloxacin* (Levaquin®) Pregnancy: C; Lactation: Unsafe **Tabs:** 250 mg, 500 mg - $$ Use with antimotility drug such as loperamide (Imodium®) if no fever or blood in stool.	**≥18 and Adult, Mild to Moderate:** 500 mg PO × 1 dose. **≥18 and Adult, Severe:** 500 mg PO Q24H × 3 days.	**Food:** May take with or without meals. Do not take within 2 hours of antacids, magnesium, calcium supplements, aluminum, sucralfate, vitamins, or minerals (iron or zinc). **Important side effects:** Photosensitivity, dizziness. **Reduce dose in renal disease (CrCl <50 mL/min).**
Azithromycin* **Alternative for children and pregnant women.** (Zithromax®) Pregnancy: B; Lactation: Unk **Tabs:** 250 mg and Z-Pak (500 mg × 1 day, then 250 mg daily × 4) **Oral Susp:** 100 mg/5 mL, 200 mg/5 mL 20-kg child - $$ Z-Pak - $$$	**Children≥ 6 months:** 5-10 mg/kg/day (max 500 mg) once daily for 5 days. **100 mg/tsp @ 10 mg/kg/day** 10 kg (22 lb) = 1 tsp (5 mL) once daily for 5 days. **200 mg/tsp @ 10 mg/kg/day** 20 kg (44 lb) = 1 tsp (5 mL) Q24H 30 kg (66 lb) = 1½ tsp (7.5 mL) Q24H 40 kg (88 lb) = 2 tsp (10 mL) Q24H ≥50 kg (110 lb) = Use adult dose. **Adult, Mild to Moderate:** 1,000 mg × 1 dose. **Adult, Severe:** Dispense one Z-Pak.	**Food:** Oral suspension should be taken 1 hour before or 2 hours after food. Tablets may be taken without regard to food. **Important side effects:** Nausea, diarrhea, elevated LFTs.
Trimethoprim/Sulfamethoxazole* (Bactrim®, Septra®) Generics available Pregnancy: C; Lactation: Unsafe	**Children:** 6-12 mg/kg/day (trimethoprim component, max 320 mg/day) in divided doses two times daily for 3-5 days. **40 mg/200 mg/5 mL @ 8 mg/kg/day**	**Food:** May take without regard to food. Encourage fluids.

(continued)

GASTROINTESTINAL – Diarrhea, Acute, Traveler's, Mild to Severe (*Shigella, E. coli, Salmonella*)

Drug, Its Forms and Dosage Increments	Children and Adult Dosages and Instructions	Information and Important Side Effects
Single Strength (SS) Tabs: 80 mg/400 mg - <$ **Double Strength (DS) Tabs:** 160 mg/800 mg - <$ **Susp:** 40 mg/200 mg/5 mL	10 kg (22 lb) 5 mL Q12H 20 kg (44 lb) 10 mL or 1 SS Tablet Q12H 30 kg (66 lb) 15 mL Q12H 1½ SS Tablet Q12H 40 kg (88 lb) 20 mL or 2 SS Tab or 1 Septra DS Q12H **Adult:** 1 DS Tab PO Q12H for 3 days.	**Important side effects:** Photosensitivity, rash. **Reduce dose in renal disease (CrCl <30 mL/min).**

GASTROINTESTINAL – Diarrhea, *Giardia* (*protozoal*)

Drug, Its Forms and Dosage Increments	Children and Adult Dosages and Instructions	Information and Important Side Effects
Metronidazole* (Flagyl®) Generics available Pregnancy: B; Lactation: Unsafe **Tabs:** 250 mg, 500 mg - <$	**Children:** 15 mg/kg/day (max 300 mg/day) in divided doses three times daily for 5-10 days. **Adult:** 250 mg three times daily for 7 days.	**Food:** Administer on empty stomach unless GI upset occurs, then with food. **Important side effects:** Dizziness, headache, confusion, seizures, nausea, metallic taste, insomnia, paresthesias. May cause Disulfiram-like reaction – avoid alcohol.

GASTROINTESTINAL – Diarrhea (*Salmonella typhi*)

Drug, Its Forms and Dosage Increments	Children and Adult Dosages and Instructions	Information and Important Side Effects
Ciprofloxacin* (Cipro®) Pregnancy: C; Lactation: Unsafe **Tabs:** 250 mg, 500 mg, 750 mg - $$$	**≥18 and Adult:** 500 mg PO twice daily for 5-7 days.	**Food:** Take on empty stomach 1 hour before or 2 hours after a meal. May take with food if it causes GI upset, but avoid large amounts of dairy products. May take 2 hours before or 6 hours after sucralfate, antacids, aluminum, magnesium, calcium, zinc, iron,

		sucralfate, vitamins, or mineral supplements. **Important side effects:** Photosensitivity, dizziness. **Reduce dose in renal disease (CrCl <50 mL/min).**
Azithromycin* (Zithromax®) Pregnancy: B; Lactation: Unk **Tabs:** 250 mg - $$	**Adult:** 1,000 mg PO once, then 500 mg PO once daily for 6 days.	**Food:** Oral suspension should be taken 1 hour before or 2 hours after food. Tablets may be taken without regard to food. **Important side effects:** Nausea, diarrhea, elevated LFTs.
Trimethoprim/Sulfamethoxazole* (Bactrim®, Septra®) Generics available Pregnancy: C; Lactation: Unsafe **Single Strength (SS) Tabs:** 80 mg/400 mg - <$ **Double Strength (DS) Tabs:** 160 mg/800 mg - <$ **Susp:** 40 mg/200 mg/5 mL *Resistance may be increasing.	**Children:** 6-12mg/kg/day (trimethoprim component, max 320 mg/day) in divided doses two time daily for 5-7 days. **40 mg/200 mg/5 mL @ 8 mg/kg/day** 10 kg (22 lb) 5 mL Q12H 20 kg (44 lb) 10 mL or 1 SS Tablet Q12H 30 kg (66 lb) 15 mL Q12H 1½ SS Tablet Q12H 40 kg (88 lb) 20 mL or 2 SS Tab or 1 Septra DS Q12H **Adult:** 1 DS tablet PO twice daily for 5-7 days.	**Food:** May take without regard to food. Encourage fluids. **Important side effects:** Photosensitivity, rash. **Reduce dose in renal disease (CrCl <30 mL/min).**

(continued)

Drug, Its Forms and Dosage Increments	Children and Adult Dosages and Instructions	Information and Important Side Effects
GASTROINTESTINAL - Diarrhea, *Staphylococcus aureus* Antibiotic treatment not recommended.		
GASTROINTESTINAL - Diarrhea, *Amebiasis*		
Metronidazole* (Flagyl®) Pregnancy: B; Lactation: Unsafe **Tabs:** 250 mg, 375 mg, 500 mg **Flagyl ER:** 750 mg - $$	**Children:** 35-50 mg/kg/day (max 750 mg/dose) in divided doses three times daily for 5-10 days. **Adult:** 750 mg three times daily for 5-10 days.	**Food:** Administer on empty stomach unless GI upset occurs, then with food. **Important side effects:** Dizziness, headache, confusion, seizures, nausea, metallic taste, insomnia, paresthesias. May cause Disulfiram-like reaction – avoid alcohol.
GASTROINTESTINAL - Diarrhea, *Campylobacter jejuni*		
Ciprofloxacin* (Cipro®) Pregnancy: C; Lactation: Unsafe **Tabs:** 250 mg, 500 mg, 750 mg - $$ *Resistance is increasing.	**≥18 and Adult:** 500 mg PO twice daily for 3-5 days.	**Food:** Take on empty stomach 1 hour before or 2 hours after a meal. May take with food if it causes GI upset, but avoid large amounts of dairy products. May take 2 hours before or 6 hours after sucralfate, antacids, aluminum, magnesium, calcium, zinc, iron, sucralfate, vitamins, or mineral supplements. **Important side effects:** Photosensitivity, dizziness. **Reduce dose in renal disease (CrCl <50 mL/min).**

Azithromycin* (Zithromax®) Pregnancy: B; Lactation: Unk **Tabs:** 250 mg - $$	**Adult:** 500 mg PO once daily for 3 days.	**Food:** Oral suspension should be taken 1 hour before or 2 hours after food. Tablets may be taken without regard to food. **Important side effects:** Nausea, diarrhea, elevated LFTs.
Erythromycin Base* (E-Mycin®, Ery-Tab®) Pregnancy: B; Lactation: Safe **Estolate:** **Tabs:** 500 mg - <$ **Caps:** 250 mg - <$ **Susp:** 125 mg/5 mL, 250 mg/5 mL - <$ **Oral Drops:** 100 mg/mL **Base:** **Tabs:** 250 mg, 333 mg, 500 mg **Caps:** 250 mg	**Children:** 30-50 mg/kg/day (max 2000 mg/day) in divided doses four times 5-7 days. **200 mg/tsp @ 50 mg/kg/day** 4-6 kg (10-15 lb) = ¼ tsp Q6H 7-11 kg (16-25 lb) = ½ tsp (2.5 mL) Q6H 11-22 kg (26-50 lb) = 1 tsp (5 mL) Q6H 23-45 kg (51-100 lb) = 1½ tsp (7.5 mL) Q6H >100 lb = Use adult dose. **Children <6 years:** 125 mg PO three times daily 10-14 days. **Adult:** 250-500 mg PO four times daily for 5-7 days.	**Food:** Take 1 hour before or 2 hours after meals. If GI upset occurs may take with food. **Important side effects:** Diarrhea, nausea, vomiting, headache, abdominal pain, dizziness, elevated LFTs, superinfection, rash, hearing loss, cardiac arrhythmias.

GASTROINTESTINAL – Diarrhea, *Clostridium difficile*

For relapses, treat again with metronidazole,possibly adding rifampin 300 mg PO Q12H × 10 days.

Metronidazole* (Flagyl®) Generics available	**Children:** 30 mg/kg/day (max 1,000 mg/day) in divided doses every 6 hours for 7-10 days.	**Food:** Administer on empty stomach unless GI upset occurs, then with food.

(continued)

Drug, Its Forms and Dosage Increments	Children and Adult Dosages and Instructions	Information and Important Side Effects
Pregnancy: B; Lactation: Unsafe **Tabs:** 250 mg, 500 mg - <$	**Adult:** 500 mg PO three times daily **or** 250 mg PO four times daily for 10-14 days.	**Important side effects:** Dizziness, headache, confusion, seizures, nausea, metallic taste, insomnia, paresthesias. Avoid alcohol.
Vancomycin* (Vancocin®) Pregnancy: C; Lactation: Unk **Caps:** 125 mg, 250 mg **Oral Sol:** 1,000 mg/20 mL or 500 mg/6 mL	**Children:** 40 mg/kg/day (max 2000 mg/day) in divided doses PO every 6 hours for 10-14 days. Usual dose 125 mg every 6 hours. **Adult:** 125-500 mg PO every 6 hours for 10-14 days. Usual dose 125 mg every 6 hours.	**Important side effects:** Adverse effects of excessive systemic levels may include ototoxicity, nephrotoxicity, hematologic effects or hypersensitivity reactions. Therapeutic drug level monitoring is rarely necessary, but might be considered for patients receiving large oral doses in a setting of severe colitis and significant renal dysfunction.

GASTROINTESTINAL – Diverticulitis (*Enterobacteriaceae*, anaerobes) **General statement:** Outpatient therapy with oral agents may be appropriate for adults with mild disease, good oral fluid intake, and a good outpatient support system. More advanced disease requires hospitalization.

Drug, Its Forms and Dosage Increments	Children and Adult Dosages and Instructions	Information and Important Side Effects
Ciprofloxacin* (Cipro®) Pregnancy: C; Lactation: Unsafe **Tabs:** 250 mg, 500 mg, 750 mg - >$$$$	**Adult:** 500 mg PO twice daily for 7-14 days. ***Use in conjunction with Metronidazole. See below.**	**Food:** Take on empty stomach 1 hour before or 2 hours after a meal. May take with food if it causes GI upset, but avoid large amounts of dairy products. May take 2 hours before or 6 hours after sucralfate, antacids, aluminum, magnesium, calcium, zinc, iron, sucralfate, vitamins, or mineral supplements.

		Important side effects: Photosensitivity, dizziness. **Reduce dose in renal disease (CrCl <50 mL/min).**
Trimethoprim/Sulfamethoxazole* (Bactrim®, Septra®) Generics available Pregnancy: C; Lactation: Unsafe **Single Strength (SS) Tabs:** 80 mg/400 mg - <$ **Double Strength (DS) Tabs:** 160 mg/800 mg - <$	**Adult:** 1 DS tablet PO twice daily for 7-14 days. *** Use in conjunction with metronidazole. See below.**	**Food:** May take without regard to food. Encourage fluids. **Important side effects:** Photosensitivity, rash. **Reduce dose in renal disease (CrCl <30 mL/min).**
Metronidazole* (Flagyl®) Generics available Pregnancy: B; Lactation: Unsafe **Tabs:** 250 mg, 500 mg - <$	**Adult:** 500 mg PO four times daily for 7-14 days. ***Use in conjunction with trimethoprim/sulfamethoxazole or ciprofloxacin. See above.**	**Food:** Administer on empty stomach unless GI upset occurs, then with food. **Important side effects:** Dizziness, headache, confusion, seizures, nausea, metallic taste, insomnia, paresthesias. Avoid alcohol. Use with caution in persons with history of seizure disorder.
Amoxicillin/clavulanate (Augmentin®) Pregnancy: B; Lactation: Unk **Q12H Formulations:** **Tabs:** 500 mg/125 mg, 875 mg/125 mg - >$$$$	**Adult:** 500 mg/125 mg PO twice daily for 7-10 days.	**Food:** Take with food to minimize diarrhea. **Important side effects:** Diarrhea. May cause nonallergic amoxicillin rash. **Use with caution in hepatic disease.** **Reduce dose in renal disease (CrCl <30 mL/min).**

(continued)

Drug, Its Forms and Dosage Increments	Children and Adult Dosages and Instructions	Information and Important Side Effects
GASTROINTESTINAL – Warts, Anogenital – External (human papilloma virus) **General statement:** Primary goal of treatment is removal of visible symptomatic warts.		
Imiquimod Cream 5% (Aldara Cream®) Pregnancy: B; Lactation: Unk **Cream 5%:** 250-mg single-use packets in box of 12 packets.	**Adult:** Apply with finger to the warts at bedtime three times per week. Gently rub in until cream is no longer visible. Leave on 6-10 hours, then gently wash area with soap and water. Continue until all warts have cleared or up to 16 weeks. Wash hands before and after application.	**Important side effects:** Itching and burning. Erythema is common. May take a rest period if needed to allow discomfort to subside.
Podofilox (Condylox®) Pregnancy: C; Lactation: Unsafe **Topical Solution 0.5%:** 3.5 mL bottle. Indicated for external genital warts only, not for perianal or mucous membrane application. **Topical Gel 0.5%:** 3.5-g tube. Indicated for external genital and perianal warts, not for mucous membrane application.	**Adults:** Apply minimal amount to cover wart with cotton-tipped applicator Q12H for 3 days, then none for 4 days. Allow to air dry before contact with opposing skin or clothing. Wash hands before and after use. Repeat weekly until no warts are seen or up to 4 weeks.	**Important side effects:** Burning, pain, itching, inflammation, erosion, bleeding. Avoid contact with eye(s). If eye(s) contact occurs, flush with water immediately and seek medical evaluation.
GENITOURINARY – Epididymitis Age <35 Years or Recent Sexual Contact (*N. gonorrhoeae, C. trachomatis*) **General statement:** Must rule out testicular torsion, a surgical emergency.		
Ceftriaxone (IM) (Rocephin®)	**Adolescents and Adult:** 250 mg IM × 1 dose.	**Important side effects:** Pain at injection site.

Drug	Dosage	Comments
Vials: 250 mg, 500 mg, 1,000 mg - $ **Vials with 2.1 mL Lidocaine for IM injection:** 500 mg, 1,000 mg	**Administer with doxycycline. See below.**	
Doxycycline* (Vibramycin®) Generics available **Caps:** 50 mg, 100 mg - <$ **Tabs:** 100 mg - <$	**Adult:** 100 mg PO twice daily for 10 days. **Administer with ceftriaxone. See above.**	**Food:** May take with food if GI upset occurs. Take 1 hour before or 2 hours after antacids, iron, milk, or other dairy products. Take with full glass of water to prevent esophagitis. **Important side effects:** Photosensitivity, use sunscreen. Esophagitis. May discolor fingernails.
Ofloxacin* (Floxin®) **Tabs:** 200 mg, 300 mg, 400 mg - >$$$$	**Adult:** 300 mg PO twice daily for 10 days.	**Food:** Take on empty stomach. Do not take within 2 hours of antacids, magnesium, calcium, zinc, iron, aluminum, sucralfate, vitamins, or mineral supplements. **Important side effects:** Nausea, photosensitivity, dizziness.

GENITOURINARY – Epididymitis Age >35 Years or No Sexual Contact (*Enterobacteriaceae*)

Drug	Dosage	Comments
Ciprofloxacin* (Cipro®) **Tabs:** 250 mg, 500 mg, 750 mg - >$$$$	**Adult:** 500 mg PO twice daily for 10-14 days.	**Food:** Take on empty stomach 1 hour before or 2 hours after a meal. May take with food if it causes GI upset, but avoid large amounts of dairy products. May take 2 hours before or 6 hours

(continued)

Drug, Its Forms and Dosage Increments	Children and Adult Dosages and Instructions	Information and Important Side Effects
		after sucralfate, antacids, aluminum, magnesium, calcium, zinc, iron, sucralfate, vitamins, or mineral supplements. **Important side effects:** Photosensitivity, dizziness. **Reduce dose in renal disease (CrCl <50 mL/min).**
Ofloxacin* (Floxin®) **Tabs:** 200 mg, 300 mg, 400 mg - >$$$$	**Adult:** 200-300 mg PO twice daily for 10 days.	**Food:** Take on empty stomach. Do not take within 2 hours of antacids, magnesium, calcium, zinc, iron, aluminum, sucralfate, vitamins, or mineral supplements. **Important side effects:** Nausea, photosensitivity, dizziness. **Reduce dose in renal disease (CrCl <50 mL/min).**

GENITOURINARY – STD, Pelvic Inflammatory Disease (*N. gonorrhoeae*, *C. trachomatis*, anaerobes, enteric gram -negative rods, *G. vaginalis*, *Streptococci*) **General statement:** Patients with pelvic inflammatory disease should be carefully evaluated to select those appropriate for outpatient therapy. Patients who do not respond within 72 hours should be reevaluated and considered for parenteral therapy.

Drug, Its Forms and Dosage Increments	Children and Adult Dosages and Instructions	Information and Important Side Effects
Ofloxacin* (Floxin®) Pregnancy: C; Lactation: Unk	**≥18 years:** 400 mg twice daily for 14 days.	**Food:** Take on empty stomach. Do not take within 2 hours of antacids, magnesium, calcium, zinc, iron,

Tabs: 200 mg, 300 mg, 400 mg - >$$$$ *** Use in conjunction with metronidazole. See below.**		aluminum, sucralfate, vitamins, or mineral supplements. **Important side effects:** Nausea, photosensitivity, dizziness. **Reduce dose in renal disease (CrCl <50 mL/min).**
Metronidazole* (Flagyl®) Generics available Pregnancy: B; Lactation: Unsafe **Tabs:** 250 mg, 500 mg - <$ ***Use in conjunction with ofloxacin. See above.**	**Adult:** 500 mg twice daily for 14 days.	**Food:** Administer on empty stomach unless GI upset occurs, then with food. **Important side effects:** Dizziness, headache, confusion, seizures, nausea, metallic taste, insomnia, paresthesias. May cause Disulfiram-like reaction – avoid alcohol.
Ceftriaxone (IM) (Rocephin®) Pregnancy: B; Lactation: Unk **Vials:** 250 mg, 500 mg, 1,000 mg - $ ***Use in conjunction with doxycycline. See below.**	**Adolescent and Adults:** 250 mg IM × 1 dose.	**Important side effects:** Pain at injection site.
Doxycycline* (Vibramycin®) Generics available Pregnancy: D; Lactation: Unsafe **Caps:** 50 mg, 100 mg - <$ **Tabs:** 100 mg ***Use in conjunction with ceftriaxone. See above.**	**Adolescent and Adults:** 100 mg PO twice daily for 14 days.	**Food:** May take with food if GI upset occurs. Take 1 hour before or 2 hours after antacids, iron, milk, or other dairy products. Take with full glass of water to prevent esophagitis. **Important side effects:** Photosensitivity, use sunscreen. Esophagitis. May discolor fingernails.

(continued)

Drug, Its Forms and Dosage Increments	Children and Adult Dosages and Instructions	Information and Important Side Effects
GENITOURINARY – Prostatitis, Acute Bacterial (*E. coli*, *Enterobacteriaceae*, *N. gonorrhoeae*, *C. trachomatis*, *Enterococci* [less commonly])		
Ciprofloxacin* (Cipro®) **Tabs:** 250 mg, 500 mg, 750 mg - >$$$$	**Adult:** 500 mg PO twice daily for 4 weeks.	**Food:** Take on empty stomach 1 hour before or 2 hours after a meal. May take with food if it causes GI upset, but avoid large amounts of dairy products. May take 2 hours before or 6 hours after sucralfate, antacids, aluminum, magnesium, calcium, zinc, iron, sucralfate, vitamins, or mineral supplements. **Important side effects:** Photosensitivity, dizziness. **Reduce dose in renal disease (CrCl <50 mL/min).**
Levofloxacin* (Levaquin®) **Tabs:** 250 mg, 500 mg - >$$$$	**Adult:** 500 mg PO daily for 4 weeks.	**Food:** May take with or without meals. Do not take within 2 hours of antacids, magnesium, calcium supplements, zinc, aluminum, sucralfate, vitamins, or minerals (iron or zinc). **Important side effects:** Photosensitivity, dizziness. **Reduce dose in renal disease (CrCl <50 mL/min).**

Ofloxacin* (Floxin®) **Tabs:** 200 mg, 300 mg, 400 mg - >$$$$	**Adult:** 400 mg PO twice daily for 4 weeks.	**Food:** Take on empty stomach. Do not take within 2 hours of antacids, magnesium, calcium, zinc, iron, aluminum, sucralfate, vitamins, or mineral supplements. **Important side effects:** Nausea, photosensitivity, dizziness. **Reduce dose in renal disease (CrCl <50 mL/min).**
Trimethoprim/ sulfamethoxazole* (Bactrim®, Septra®) Generics available **Single Strength (SS) Tabs:** 80 mg/400 mg - <$ **Double Strength (DS) Tabs:** 160 mg/800 mg - <$	**Adult:** 1 DS tablet PO twice daily for 4 weeks.	**Food:** May take without regard to food. Encourage fluids. **Important side effects:** Photosensitivity, rash. **Reduce dose in renal disease (CrCl <30 mL/min).**

GENITOURINARY – Prostatitis, Chronic Bacterial (*Enterobacteriaceae*, *Enterococci*) Most cases of "prostatitis" are not caused by bacterial infection. Chronic prostatitis is characterized by relapsing bacteriuria.

Ciprofloxacin* (Cipro®) **Tabs:** 250 mg, 500 mg, 750 mg - >$$$$	**Adult:** 500 mg PO twice daily for 6-12 weeks.	**Food:** Take on empty stomach 1 hour before or 2 hours after a meal. May take with food if it causes GI upset, but avoid large amounts of dairy products. May take 2 hours before or 6 hours after sucralfate, antacids, aluminum, *(continued)*

Drug, Its Forms and Dosage Increments	Children and Adult Dosages and Instructions	Information and Important Side Effects
		magnesium, calcium, zinc, iron, sucralfate, vitamins, or mineral supplements. **Important side effects:** Photosensitivity, dizziness. **Reduce dose in renal disease (CrCl <50 mL/min).**
Levofloxacin* (Levaquin®) **Tabs:** 250 mg, 500 mg - >$$$$	**≥18 and Adult:** 500 mg PO daily for 6-12 weeks.	**Food:** May take with or without meals. Do not take within 2 hours of antacids, magnesium, calcium supplements, zinc, aluminum, sucralfate, vitamins, or minerals (iron or zinc). **Important side effects:** Photosensitivity, dizziness. **Reduce dose in renal disease (CrCl <50 mL/min).**
Ofloxacin* (Floxin®) **Tabs:** 200 mg, 300 mg, 400 mg - >$$$$	**Adult:** 400 mg PO twice daily for 6-12 weeks.	**Food:** Take on empty stomach. Do not take within 2 hours of antacids, magnesium, calcium, zinc, iron, aluminum, sucralfate, vitamins, or mineral supplements. **Important side effects:** Nausea, photosensitivity, dizziness. **Reduce dose in renal disease (CrCl <50 mL/min).**

Doxycycline* (Vibramycin®) Generics available **Caps:** 50 mg, 100 mg - <$-$ **Tabs:** 100 mg	**Adult:** 100 mg PO twice daily for 6-12 weeks.	**Food:** May take with food if GI upset occurs. Take 1 hour before or 2 hours after antacids, iron, milk, or other dairy products. Take with full glass of water to prevent esophagitis. **Important side effects:** Photosensitivity, use sunscreen. Esophagitis. May discolor fingernails.
Trimethoprim/Sulfamethoxazole* (Bactrim®, Septra®) Generics available **Single Strength (SS)** **Tabs:** 80 mg/400 mg - <$ **Double Strength (DS)** **Tabs:** 160 mg/800 mg - <$	**Adult:** 1 DS tablet PO twice daily for 6-12 weeks.	**Food:** May take without regard to food. **Encourage fluids.** **Important side effects:** Photosensitivity, rash. **Reduce dose in renal disease (CrCl <30 mL/min).**

GENITOURINARY – UTI – Adult – Acute Uncomplicated Cystitis (*E. coli*, *S. saprophyticus*, other enterobacteria, *Proteus*, *Enterococci*)

Ciprofloxacin* (Cipro®) Pregnancy: C; Lactation: Unsafe **Tabs:** 100 mg, 250 mg, 500 mg - >$$$$	**≥18 and Adult:** **Young women:** 100-250 mg twice daily for 3 days. **Young men and older men without evidence of prostatitis:** 250-500 mg twice daily for 7-14 days.	**Food:** Take on empty stomach 1 hour before or 2 hours after a meal. May take with food if it causes GI upset, but avoid large amounts of dairy products. May take 2 hours before or 6 hours after sucralfate, antacids, aluminum, magnesium, calcium, zinc, iron, sucralfate, vitamins, or mineral supplements.

(continued)

Drug, Its Forms and Dosage Increments	Children and Adult Dosages and Instructions	Information and Important Side Effects
		Important side effects: Photosensitivity, dizziness. **Reduce dose in renal disease (CrCl <50 mL/min).**
Levofloxacin* (Levaquin®) Pregnancy: C; Lactation: Unsafe **Tabs:** 250 mg, 500 mg - >$$$$	**≥18 and Adult:** **Young women:** 250 mg daily for 3 days. **Young men and older men without evidence of prostatitis:** 250 mg daily for 7-14 days.	**Food:** May take with or without meals. Do not take within 2 hours of antacids, magnesium, calcium supplements, zinc, aluminum, sucralfate, vitamins, or minerals (iron or zinc). **Important side effects:** Photosensitivity, dizziness. **Reduce dose in renal disease (CrCl <50 mL/min).**
Nitrofurantoin* (Macrodantin®, Macrobid®) Generics available Pregnancy: B; (Do not use at term or in labor) Lactation: Unsafe **Caps:** 25 mg, 50 mg, 100 mg - <$ **Oral Susp:** 25 mg/5 mL - $$ **Macrobid (extended release):** 100 mg Q12H - $	**Young women:** 50-100 mg PO every 6 hours for 3 days or Macrobid 100 mg PO every 12 hours for 3 days. **Young men and older men without evidence of prostatitis:** Not recommended for use in men due to poor tissue penetration.	**Food:** Take with food or milk. **Important side effects:** Nausea, vomiting, darkening of the urine, headache, hepatitis, peripheral neuropathy. **Ineffective if CrCl ≤40 mL/min**

**E. coli* resistance increasing and may be significant. Not advocated as first-line therapy.		
Trimethoprim/Sulfamethoxazole* (Bactrim®, Septra®) Generics available Pregnancy: C; Lactation: Unsafe **Single strength (SS) Tabs:** 80 mg/400 mg - <$ **Double Strength (DS) Tabs:** 160 mg/800 mg - <$ **Oral Susp:** 40 mg/200 mg/5 mL **E. coli* resistance may be 15-20% and may require alternative therapy in many locales.	**Young women:** 1 DS tablet twice daily for 3 days. **Young men and older men without evidence of prostatitis:** 1 DS tablet twice daily for 7-14 days.	**Food:** May take without regard to food. Encourage fluids. **Important side effects:** Photosensitivity, rash. **Reduce dose in renal disease (CrCl <30 mL/min).**

GENITOURINARY – UTI – Child – Acute Uncomplicated Cystitis (*E. coli, Enterobacter, Klebsiella*)

Amoxicillin/clavulanate (Augmentin®) **Q12H Formulations:** **Tabs:** 500 mg/125 mg, 875 mg/125 mg **Chewable Tabs:** 200 mg/28.5 mg, 400 mg/57 mg **Oral Susp:** 200 mg/28.5 mg/5 mL, 400 mg/57 mg/5 mL Child - $$$	**Children:** 40-50 mg amoxicillin component/kg/day (max 1600 mg/day) in divided doses two or three times daily for 7 days. **Q12H using 200 mg/5 mL susp @ 45 mg/kg/day** 9 kg (20 lb) = 1 tsp (5 mL) Q12H 13 kg (29 lb) = 1½ tsp (7.5 mL) Q12H 18 kg (40 lb) = 2 tsp (10 mL) Q12H	**Food:** Take with food to reduce diarrhea. **Important side effects:** Diarrhea (common), nausea, rash. **Use with caution in hepatic disease.** **Reduce dose in renal disease (CrCl <30 mL/min).**

(continued)

Drug, Its Forms and Dosage Increments	Children and Adult Dosages and Instructions	Information and Important Side Effects
	Q12H using 400 mg/5 mL susp @ 45 mg/kg/day 18 kg (40 lb) = 1 tsp (5 mL) Q12H 27 kg (59 lb) = 1½ tsp (7.5 mL) Q12H 35 kg (77 lb) = 2 tsp (10 mL) Q12H >40 kg = Use adult dose (max 875 mg Q12H). Note: Q12H dosing may improve compliance compared to Q8H dosing.	
Cefixime (Suprax®) **Tabs:** 200 mg, 400 mg **Oral Susp:** 100 mg/5 mL - $$$$	**Children:** 8 mg/kg/day (max 400 mg/day) as single dose or divided twice daily for 7 days. **100 mg/5 mL @ 8 mg/kg/day** 12.5 kg (27.5 lb) = ½ tsp (2.5 mL) Q12H 19 kg (42 lb) = ¾ tsp Q12H 25 kg (55 lb) = 1 tsp (5 mL) Q12H 38 kg (77 lb) = 1½ (7.5 mL) Q12H >50 kg (110 lb) = Use adult dose.	**Food:** May administer on empty stomach. May administer with food to reduce GI distress. **Important side effects:** Nausea, diarrhea.
Cefpodoxime (Vantin®) **Tabs:** 100 mg - $$$ 200 mg - $$$ **Granules for Oral Suspension:** 50 mg/5 mL	**Children ≥5 months to 12 years:** 10 mg/kg/day (max 400 mg/day) in one or two divided doses for 7 days. **50 mg/5 mL @ 10 mg/kg/day** 10 kg (22 lb) = 1 tsp (5 mL) Q12H 15 kg (33 lb) = 1½ tsp (7.5 mL) Q12H	**Food:** Take tablet with food. Suspension may be taken without regard to food. **Important side effects:** Nausea, vomiting, rash, diarrhea, elevated LFTs. **Caution:** Use with caution in patients with history of seizures.

(50, 75, 100 mL) 100 mL - $$ 100 mg/5 mL (50, 75, 100 mL) 100 mL - $$$$	**100 mg/5 mL @10 mg/kg/day** 15 kg (33 lb) = ¾ tsp Q12H 20 kg (44 lb) = 1 tsp (5 mL) Q12H 30 kg (66 lb) = 1½ tsp (7.5 mL) Q12H 40 kg (88 lb) = Use adult dose.	**Reduce dose in renal disease.** CrCl <30 mL/min increase dosing interval to once daily.
Cefprozil (Cefzil®) **Tabs:** 250 mg - $$ 500 mg - $$$$ **Powder for Oral Suspension:** 125 mg/5 mL (50, 75, 100 mL) 100 mL - $$ 250 mg/5 mL (50, 75, 100 mL) 100 mL - $$$$	**Children ≥6 months to 12 years:** 7.5-15 mg/kg/day in divided doses 2 times daily (max 1,000 mg/day) **250 mg/5 mL @ 30 mg/kg/day** 9.1 kg (20 lb) = ½ tsp (2.5 mL) Q12H 13.6 kg (30 lb) = ¾ tsp Q12H 18.2 kg (40 lb) = 1 tsp (5 mL) Q12H 27 kg (60 lb) = 1½ tsp (7.5 mL) Q12H 31 kg (70 lb) = Use adult dose.	**Food:** May be taken without regard to food. May take with food to reduce GI upset. **Important side effects:** Nausea, vomiting, rash, diarrhea, elevated LFTs. **Caution:** Use with caution in patients with history of seizures. **Reduce dose in renal disease:** CrCl <30 mL/min administer 50% of usual dose at standard dosing interval.
Nitrofurantoin* (Macrodantin®, Macrobid®) Generics available **Caps:** 25 mg, 50 mg, 100 mg - <$ **Oral Susp:** 25 mg/5 mL - $$ **Macrobid (extended release):** 100 mg Q12H - $ **E. coli* resistance increasing and may be significant. Not advocated as first-line therapy.	**Children ≥1 month:** 5-7 mg/kg/day (max 400 mg/day) in divided doses every 6 hours for 7 days. **25 mg/5 mL @ 5 mg/kg/day** 10 kg (22 lb) = ½ tsp (2.5 mL) Q6H 20 kg (44 lb) = 1 tsp (5 mL) Q6H 30 kg (66 lb) = 1½ tsp (7.5 mL) Q6H 40 kg (88 lb) = 2 tsp (10 mL) Q6H	**Food:** Take with food or milk. **Important side effects:** Nausea, vomiting, darkening of the urine, headache, hepatitis, peripheral neuropathy. **Ineffective if CrCl ≤40 mL/min**

(continued)

GENITOURINARY – UTI – Child – Acute Uncomplicated Cystitis (*E. coli, Enterobacter, Klebsiella*)

Drug, Its Forms and Dosage Increments	Children and Adult Dosages and Instructions	Information and Important Side Effects
Trimethoprim/ Sulfamethoxazole* (Bactrim®, Septra®) Generics available **Single strength (SS) Tabs:** 80 mg/400 mg - <$ **Double Strength (DS) Tabs:** 160 mg/800 mg - <$ **Oral Susp:** 40 mg/200 mg/5 mL - $ **E. coli* resistance may be 15-20% and may require alternative therapy in many locales.	**Children ≥ 2 months:** 6-12 mg/kg/day TMP component (max 320 mg/day) in divided doses twice daily for 7 days. **40 mg/200 mg/5 mL @ 6-12 mg/kg/day** 10 kg (22 lb) = 1 tsp (5 mL) Q12H 20 kg (44 lb) = 2 tsp (10 mL) or 1 SS tab Q12H 30 kg (66 lb) = 3 tsp (15 mL) or 1½ SS tab Q12H 40 kg (88 lb) = 4 tsp (20 mL) or 2 SS tabs **or** 1 DS Tab Q12H for 3-5 days	**Food:** May take without regard to food. Encourage fluids. **Important side effects:** Photosensitivity, rash. **Reduce dose in renal disease (CrCl <30 mL/min).**

GENITOURINARY – UTI – Child – Acute Pyelonephritis

Note: May consider outpatient therapy for child ≥3 months, who: appears well, is not vomiting, tolerates fluids well, and for whom good compliance and follow-up are likely. May initiate in-office therapy with IM ceftriaxone.

Drug, Its Forms and Dosage Increments	Children and Adult Dosages and Instructions	Information and Important Side Effects
Ceftriaxone (Rocephin®) **Powder for IM or IV injection:** 250 mg - $, 500 mg - $$, 1,000 mg - $$	**Children:** 50-75 mg/kg/day (max 1,000 mg) IM in a single daily dose for 1-2 days followed by oral therapy with one of the agent listed below.	**Important side effects:** Rash, diarrhea, elevated LFTs. Reduce dose in patients with combined liver disease and significant renal disease. **Caution:** Use cautiously in patients with history of seizures. Use with caution in patients with history of biliary disease.

Cefixime (Suprax®) **Tabs:** 200 mg, 400 mg **Oral Susp:** 100 mg/5 mL - $$$$	**Children:** 8 mg/kg/day (max 400 mg/day) as single dose or divided twice daily for 10-14 days. May initiate therapy with cefixime @ 16mg/kg/day (max 400 mg) twice daily for the fist day as an alternative to ceftriaxone. **100 mg/5 mL @ 8 mg/kg/day** 12.5 kg (27.5 lb) = ½ tsp (2.5 mL) Q12H 19 kg (42 lb) = ¾ tsp Q12H 25 kg (55 lb) = 1 tsp (5 mL) Q12H 38 kg (77 lb) = 1½ (7.5 mL) Q12H >50 kg (110 lb) = Use adult dose.	**Food:** May administer on empty stomach. May administer with food to reduce GI distress. **Important side effects:** Nausea, diarrhea.
Cefpodoxime (Vantin®) **Tabs:** 100 mg 200 mg **Granules for Oral Suspension:** 50 mg/5 mL (50, 75, 100 mL) 100 mL - $$ 100 mg/5 mL (50, 75, 100 mL) 100 mL - $$$	**Children ≥5 months to 12 years:** 10 mg/kg/day (max 400 mg/day) in one or two divided doses for 10-14 days. **50 mg/5 mL @ 10 mg/kg/day** 10 kg (22 lb) = 1 tsp (5 mL) Q12H 15 kg (33 lb) = 1½ tsp (7.5 mL) Q12H **100 mg/5 mL @10 mg/kg/day** 15 kg (33 lb) = ¾ tsp Q12H 20 kg (44 lb) = 1 tsp (5 mL) Q12H 30 kg (66 lb) = 1½ tsp (7.5 mL) Q12H 40 kg (88 lb) = Use adult dose.	**Food:** Take tablet with food. Suspension may be taken without regard to food. **Important side effects:** Nausea, vomiting, rash, diarrhea, elevated LFTs. **Caution:** Use with caution in patients with history of seizures. **Reduce dose in renal disease.** CrCl <30 mL/min increase dosing interval to once daily.
Cefprozil (Cefzil®)	**Children ≥6 months to 12 years:** 7.5-15 mg/kg/day in divided doses 2 times daily (max 1,000 mg/day)	**Food:** May be taken without regard to food. May take with food to reduce GI upset.

(continued)

Drug, Its Forms and Dosage Increments	Children and Adult Dosages and Instructions	Information and Important Side Effects
Tabs: 250 mg 500 mg **Powder for Oral Suspension:** 125 mg/5 mL (50, 75, 100 mL) 100 mL - $$ 250 mg/5 mL (50, 75, 100 mL) 100 mL - $$$$	**250 mg/5 mL @ 30 mg/kg/day** 9.1 kg (20 lb) = ½ tsp (2.5 mL) Q12H 13.6 kg (30 lb) = ¾ tsp Q12H 18.2 kg (40 lb) = 1 tsp (5 mL) Q12H 27 kg (60 lb) = 1½ tsp (7.5 mL) Q12H 31 kg (70 lb) = Use adult dose.	**Important side effects:** Nausea, vomiting, rash, diarrhea, elevated LFTs. **Caution:** Use with caution in patients with history of seizures. **Reduce dose in renal disease:** CrCl <30 mL/min administer 50% of usual dose at standard dosing interval.
Trimethoprim/Sulfamethoxazole* (Bactrim®, Septra®) Generics available **Single strength (SS) Tabs:** 80 mg/400 mg - <$ **Double Strength (DS) Tabs:** 160 mg/800 mg - <$ **Oral Susp:** 40 mg/200 mg/5 mL - $ **E. coli* resistance may be 15-20% and may require alternative therapy in many locales.	**Children ≥2 months:** 6-12mg/kg/day TMP component (max 320 mg/day) in divided doses twice daily for 10-14 days. **40 mg/200 mg/5 mL @ 6-12mg/kg/day** 10 kg (22 lb) = 1 tsp (5 mL) Q12H 20 kg (44 lb) = 2 tsp (10 mL) or 1 SS Tab Q12H 30 kg (66 lb) = 3 tsp (15 mL) or 1½ SS Tab Q12H 40 kg (88 lb) = 4 tsp (20 mL) or 2 SS Tabs or 1 DS Tab Q12H for 3-5 days.	**Food:** May take without regard to food. Encourage fluids. **Important side effects:** Photosensitivity, rash. **Reduce dose in renal disease (CrCl <30 mL/min).**
Amoxicillin/clavulanate (Augmentin®)	**Children:** 40-50 mg amoxicillin component/kg/day (max 1600 mg/day) in	**Food:** Take with food to reduce diarrhea.

Q12H Formulations:
Tabs: 500 mg/125 mg, 875 mg/125 mg
Chewable Tabs:
200 mg/28.5 mg, 400 mg/57 mg
Oral Susp:
200 mg/28.5 mg/5 mL,
400 mg/57 mg/5 mL
Child - $$$

divided doses two or three times daily for 10-14 days.

Q12H using 200 mg/5 mL susp @ 45 mg/kg/day
9 kg (20 lb) = 1 tsp (5 mL) Q12H
13 kg (29 lb) = 1½ tsp (7.5 mL) Q12H
18 kg (40 lb) = 2 tsp (10 mL) Q12H

Q12H using 400 mg/5 mL susp @ 45 mg/kg/day
18 kg (40 lb) = 1 tsp (5 mL) Q12H
27 kg (59 lb) = 1½ tsp (7.5 mL) Q12H
35 kg (77 lb) = 2 tsp (10 mL) Q12H
>40 kg = Use adult dose (max 875 mg Q12H)

Important side effects: Diarrhea (common), nausea, rash.
Use with caution in hepatic disease.
Reduce dose in renal disease (CrCl <30 mL/min).

GENITOURINARY – UTI – Pregnant Woman, Asymptomatic Bacteriuria or Uncomplicated Cystitis

Amoxicillin
(Amoxil®)
Generics available
Pregnancy: B; Lactation: Unsafe
Caps: 250 mg, 500 mg - <$
Tabs: 500 mg, 875 mg - <$
E. coli resistance increasing.

Adolescent and Adult: 500 mg every 8 hours for 7 days.

Food: With or without meals.
Important side effects: Diarrhea and nausea. May cause nonallergic maculopapular rash.
Reduce dose in renal disease (CrCl <30 mL/min).

(continued)

Drug, Its Forms and Dosage Increments	Children and Adult Dosages and Instructions	Information and Important Side Effects
Cephalexin (Keflex®) Generics available Pregnancy: B; Lactation: Unk **Tabs:** 250 mg, 500 mg, 1 g - $$ **Caps:** 250 mg, 500 mg - <$	**Adolescent and Adult:** 500 mg every 6 hours for 7 days.	**Food:** May take with food if GI upset occurs. **Important side effects:** GI upset, diarrhea. **Reduce dose in renal disease (CrCl <40 mL/min).**
Trimethoprim/ sulfamethoxazole* (Bactrim®, Septra®) Generics available Pregnancy: C; Lactation: Unsafe **Single strength (SS) Tabs:** 80 mg/400 mg - <$ **Double Strength (DS) Tabs:** 160 mg/800 mg - $ **E. coli* resistance may be 15-20% and increasing. * Avoid using near term (within 2 weeks of delivery).	**Adolescent and Adult:** 1 DS tablet twice daily for 7 days.	**Food:** May take without regard to food. Encourage fluids. **Important side effects:** Photosensitivity, rash. **Reduce dose in renal disease (CrCl <30 mL/min).**

GENITOURINARY – UTI – Fungal **General statement:** Rule out systemic fungal infection. Consider removing urinary catheter, discontinuing any antibiotics, reducing steroid therapy, and controlling hyperglycemia.

Fluconazole* (Diflucan®)	**Adult:** 100 mg PO daily for 7-10 days.	**Food:** May be taken without regard to food.

Pregnancy: C; Lactation: Unsafe **Tabs**: 50 mg, 100 mg, 150 mg, 200 mg - $$$->$$$$		**Important side effects:** Advise patient to report any signs of liver failure: anorexia, nausea, vomiting, RUQ discomfort, jaundice, ascites. Potentially significant drug interactions; consult a pharmacist.

GENITOURINARY – UTI – Adult – Pyelonephritis Acute-Uncomplicated

Amoxicillin/clavulanate (Augmentin®) Pregnancy: B; Lactation: Unk **Q12H Formulations:** **Tabs:** 500 mg, 875 mg Child - $$$ Adult - >$$$$	**Adult:** 500-875 mg twice daily for 14 days. Note: Q12H dosing may improve compliance compared to Q8H dosing.	**Food:** Take with meals to reduce diarrhea. **Important side effects:** Diarrhea (take with food). May cause nonallergic amoxicillin rash. **Reduce dose in renal disease (CrCl <30 mL/min).**
<u>**Ciprofloxacin**</u>* (Cipro®) Pregnancy: C; Lactation: Unsafe **Tabs:** 250 mg, 500 mg, 750 mg - >$$$$	**≥18 and Adult:** 250-500 mg twice daily for 10-14 days.	**Food:** Take on empty stomach 1 hour before or 2 hours after a meal. May take with food if it causes GI upset, but avoid large amounts of dairy products. May take 2 hours before or 6 hours after sucralfate, antacids, aluminum, magnesium, calcium, zinc, iron, sucralfate, vitamins, or mineral supplements. **Important side effects:** Photosensitivity, dizziness.

(continued)

Drug, Its Forms and Dosage Increments	Children and Adult Dosages and Instructions	Information and Important Side Effects
		Reduce dose in renal disease (CrCl <50 mL/min).
Levofloxacin* (Levaquin®) Pregnancy: C; Lactation: Unsafe **Tabs:** 250 mg, 500 mg - >$$$$	**≥18 and Adult:** 250-500 mg daily for 10-14 days.	**Food:** May take with or without meals. Do not take within 2 hours of antacids, magnesium, calcium supplements, zinc, aluminum, sucralfate, vitamins, or minerals (iron or zinc). **Important side effects:** Photosensitivity, dizziness. **Reduce dose in renal disease (CrCl <50 mL/min).**
Trimethoprim/Sulfamethoxazole* (Bactrim®, Septra®) Generics available Pregnancy: C; Lactation: Unsafe **Single Strength (SS) Tabs:** 80 mg/400 mg - <$ **Double Strength (DS) Tabs:** 160 mg/800 mg - <$	**Adult:** 1 DS Tablet PO twice daily for 14 days.	**Food:** May take without regard to food. Encourage fluids. **Important side effects:** Photosensitivity, rash. **Reduce dose in renal disease (CrCl <30 mL/min).**

GENITOURINARY – UTI – Prophylaxis for recurrent UTIs (re-infections)

Drug, Its Forms and Dosage Increments	Children and Adult Dosages and Instructions	Information and Important Side Effects
Cephalexin (Keflex®) Generics available Pregnancy: B; Lactation: Unk	**Children:** 10 mg/kg (max 500 mg) every night at bedtime for 6 months. **Adult:** 500 mg every night at bedtime for 6 months.	**Food:** Take 1 hour before or 2 hours after meals. May take with food if GI upset occurs.

Tabs: 250 mg, 500 mg, 1 g - $$$ **Caps:** 250 mg, 500 mg - <$ **Oral Susp:** 125 mg/5 mL, 250 mg/5 mL - <$		**Important side effects:** GI upset, diarrhea.
Nitrofurantoin* (Macrodantin®) Generics available Pregnancy: B; (Not at term or in labor) Lactation: Unsafe **Caps:** 25 mg, 50 mg, 100 mg - <$ **Oral Susp:** 25 mg/5 mL - $$ **Macrobid (extended release):** 100 mg Q12H - $	**Children:** 1-2 mg/kg/day (max 100 mg) every night at bedtime for 6 months. **1-2 mg/kg/day** 10 kg (22 lb) = ½ tsp (2.5 mL) QHS 20 kg (44 lb) = 1 tsp (5 mL) QHS 30 kg (66 lb) = 1½ tsp (7.5 mL) QHS 40 kg (88 lb) = 2 tsp (10 mL) QHS **Adult:** 50-100 mg every night at bedtime for 6 months.	**Food:** Take with food or milk. **Important side effects:** Nausea, vomiting, darkening of the urine, headache, hepatitis, peripheral neuropathy.
<u>**Sulfamethoxazole**</u>*/ **Trimethoprim** (Bactrim®, Septra®) Generics available Pregnancy: C; Lactation: Unsafe **Single Strength (SS) Tabs:** 80 mg/400 mg - <$ **Double Strength (DS) Tabs:** 160 mg/800 mg - <$ **Oral Susp:** 40 mg/200 mg/5 mL - <$	**Children ≥2 months:** 2mg/kg TMP component every night **OR** 5 mg/kg TMP component twice a week at bedtime for 6 months. **Adult:** 1 SS or 1 DS Tablet at bedtime for 6 months.	**Food:** May take without regard to food. Encourage fluids. **Important side effects:** Photosensitivity, rash. **Reduce dose in renal disease (CrCl <30 mL/min).**

(continued)

Drug, Its Forms and Dosage Increments	Children and Adult Dosages and Instructions	Information and Important Side Effects
GENITOURINARY – Balanitis (Group B *Streptococcus, Staphylococci*) Genital cleansing and hygiene important. May be more severe in diabetic patients. May require urologic consultation for circumcision.		
Bacitracin (OTC)* (Baciguent®) Generics available **Ointment:** 500 U/g (1 g, 15 g, 30 g)	**Adult:** Apply four times daily until resolved.	**Important side effects:** May cause rash or itching.
GENITOURINARY – Balanitis, Fungal (*Candida sp.*)		
Clotrimazole (OTC)* (Lotrimin®, Mycelex®, Fungoid®) Generics available **Cream 1%:** 30 g **Lotion 1%:** 30 mL	**Adult:** Apply to affected area after washing and drying twice daily until resolved.	
Nystatin* (Mycostatin®, Nilstat®) Generics available **Cream:** 15 g, 30 g **Ointment:** 15 g, 30 g	**Adult:** Apply to affected area after washing and drying two to four times daily until resolved.	**Important side effects:** Contact dermatitis.
Fluconazole* (Diflucan®) **Tabs:** 50 mg, 100 mg, 150 mg, 200 mg - >$$$$	**Adult:** 100-150 mg PO once.	**Food:** May be taken without regard to food. **Important side effects:** Nausea, dizziness, hepatitis, rash. Notify doctor if you develop rash, unusual bleeding, bruising, yellow skin or eye(s), nausea, or GI pain.

GENITOURINARY – Balanitis, Resistant to Topical Therapy

Drug	Dosage	Comments
Ciprofloxacin* Cipro® **Tabs:** 250 mg, 500 mg, 750 mg - >$$$$	**Adult:** 500 mg PO twice daily for 10 days.	**Food:** Take on empty stomach 1 hour before or 2 hours after a meal. May take with food if it causes GI upset, but avoid large amounts of dairy products. May take 2 hours before or 6 hours after sucralfate, antacids, aluminum, magnesium, calcium, zinc, iron, sucralfate, vitamins, or mineral supplements. **Important side effects:** Photosensitivity, dizziness. **Reduce dose in renal disease (CrCl <50 mL/min).**

GENITOURINARY – Bacterial Vaginosis (Anaerobes, *Gardnerella vaginalis*, *Mycoplasma hominis*, polymicrobial)

Drug	Dosage	Comments
Metronidazole* (Flagyl®) Generics available Pregnancy: B; Lactation: Unsafe **Tabs:** 250 mg, 500 mg - <$	**Adult:** 500 mg twice daily for 7 days **or** 2 g given as a one time dose. (2-g dosing may be less effective than the 7-day regimen.)	**Food:** Administer on empty stomach unless GI upset occurs, then with food. **Important side effects:** Dizziness, headache, confusion, seizures, nausea, metallic taste, insomnia, paresthesias. May cause Disulfiram-like reaction – avoid alcohol.
Clindamycin Vaginal Cream* (Cleocin®) Pregnancy: B; Lactation: Unknown	**Adolescent and Adult:** Insert one applicator (5 g) intravaginally each night at bedtime for 7 days.	**Important side effects: May weaken latex condoms or diaphragms. Advise**

(continued)

Drug, Its Forms and Dosage Increments	Children and Adult Dosages and Instructions	Information and Important Side Effects
Vaginal Cream 2%: 40 g		**patient not to engage in vaginal intercourse while using this product.**
Metronidazole gel* (MetroGel®-Vaginal) Pregnancy: B; Lactation: Unk **Gel, vaginal 0.75%:** 70 g	**Adult:** Insert one applicator (5 g) intravaginally twice daily for 5 days.	
Clindamycin* (Cleocin®) Generics available Pregnancy: B; Lactation: Unk **Caps:** 150 mg - $, 300 mg - $$$	**Adult:** 300 mg twice daily for 7 days. ***May cause severe colitis.** Encourage patient to report severe, persistent, or bloody diarrhea.	**Food:** May administer without regard to food. Take with full glass of water to prevent esophagitis. **Important side effects:** Diarrhea (may be severe), esophagitis.

GENITOURINARY – Bacterial Vaginosis, Pregnancy (Anaerobes, *Gardnerella vaginalis, Mycoplasma hominis*, polymicrobial)

Drug, Its Forms and Dosage Increments	Children and Adult Dosages and Instructions	Information and Important Side Effects
Metronidazole* (Flagyl®) Generics available Pregnancy: B; Lactation: Unsafe **Tabs:** 250 mg, 500 mg - <$	**Adult:** 250 mg PO three times daily for 7 days **or** 2 g once. (2-g dosing may be less effective than the 7 day regimen).	**Food:** Administer on empty stomach unless GI upset occurs, then with food. **Important side effects:** Dizziness, headache, confusion, seizures, nausea, metallic taste, insomnia, paresthesias. May cause disulfiram-like reaction—avoid alcohol.
Clindamycin* (Cleocin®) Generics available	**Adult:** 300 mg PO twice daily for 7 days.	**Food:** May administer without regard to food. Take with full glass of water to prevent esophagitis.

Pregnancy: B; Lactation: Unknown **Caps:** 150 mg - \$, 300 mg - \$\$\$	***May cause severe colitis.** Encourage patient to report severe, persistent, or bloody diarrhea.	**Important side effects:** Diarrhea (may be severe), esophagitis.

GENITOURINARY – Vulvovaginal Candidiasis (*Candida albicans, Torulopsis sp.*)

Miconazole* (OTC) (Monistat Vaginal®, Femizol-M®) Generics available Pregnancy: C; Lactation: Unknown **Vaginal Products:** **Suppository:** 100 mg (7's), 200 mg (3's) **Cream with applicator 2%:** 45 g	**Adolescent and Adult:** 1 applicator vaginally QHS × 7 days **or** 100-mg vaginal suppository QHS × 7 days **or** 200-mg vaginal suppository QHS × 3 days.	Remain lying down for 30 minutes after application. Avoid intercourse during therapy. Do not use tampons until therapy is complete. Cream or vaginal suppositories may weaken latex condoms and diaphragms. Avoid use during first trimester of pregnancy.
Clotrimazole* (Mycelex-G®, Gyne-Lotrimin®) Generics available Pregnancy: B; Lactation: Unknown **Vaginal Products:** **Tablets:** 100 mg (7's), 500 mg (1's) **Cream with applicator 1% (OTC):** 45 g, 90 g	**Adolescent and Adult:** 1 applicator vaginally QHS × 7-14 days **or** 100-mg vaginal tablets QHS × 7 days **or** 2 × 100 mg vaginal tablets QHS × 3 days **or** 500-mg vaginal tablet QHS once.	Remain lying down for 30 minutes after application. Avoid intercourse during therapy. Do not use tampons until therapy is complete. Cream or vaginal tablets may weaken latex condoms and diaphragms.
Nystatin Vaginal Tablet* **May be less effective than topical azoles.** (Mycostatin®) Pregnancy: B; Lactation: Safe **Vaginal tablet 100,000 U:** 15's and 30's	**Adolescent and Adult:** 1 tablet vaginally QHS × 14 days.	Remain lying down for 30 minutes after application.

(continued)

Drug, Its Forms and Dosage Increments	Children and Adult Dosages and Instructions	Information and Important Side Effects
Fluconazole* (Diflucan®) Pregnancy: C; Lactation: Unsafe **Tabs:** 50 mg, 100 mg, 150 mg - >$$$$	**Adolescent and Adult:** 150 mg PO × 1 dose.	**Food:** May be taken without regard to food. **Important side effects:** Nausea, dizziness, rash.

GENITOURINARY – Vulvovaginal Candidiasis, Pregnancy (*Candida albicans, Torulopsis sp.*)

Drug, Its Forms and Dosage Increments	Children and Adult Dosages and Instructions	Information and Important Side Effects
Clotrimazole* (Mycelex-G®, Gyne-Lotrimin®) Generics available Pregnancy: B; Lactation: Unknown **Vaginal Products:** **Tablets:** 100 mg (7's), 500 mg (1's) **Cream with applicator 1% (OTC):** 45 g, 90 g	**Adolescent and Adult:** 1 applicator vaginally QHS × 7-14 days **or** 100-mg vaginal tablets QHS × 7 days **or** 2 × 100 mg vaginal tablets QHS × 3 days **or** 500-mg vaginal tablet QHS once.	Remain lying down for 30 minutes after application. Avoid intercourse during therapy. Do not use tampons until therapy is complete. Cream or vaginal tablets may weaken latex condoms.
Miconazole* (OTC) (Monistat Vaginal®) Generics available Pregnancy: C; Lactation: Unknown **Vaginal Products:** **Suppository:** 100 mg (7's), 200 mg (3's) **Cream with applicator 2%:** 45 g	**Adolescent and Adult:** 1 applicator vaginally QHS × 7 days **or** 100-mg vaginal suppository QHS × 7 days **or** 200-mg vaginal suppository QHS × 3 days.	Remain lying down for 30 minutes after application. Avoid intercourse during therapy. Do not use tampons until therapy is complete. Cream or vaginal suppositories may weaken latex condoms and diaphragms. Avoid use during first trimester of pregnancy.

GENITOURINARY – STD, Chancroid (*H. ducreyi*)

<table>
<tr>
<td>Azithromycin*
(Zithromax®)
Pregnancy: B; Lactation: Unk
Tabs: 250 mg - $$
<b>Powder for Oral Suspension:</b> 1 g - $$</td>
<td>Adolescent and Adult: 1 g × 1 dose.</td>
<td>Food: 1 g powder packet for oral suspension and tablets may be taken without regard to food.
Important side effects: Nausea, diarrhea, elevated LFTs.</td>
</tr>
<tr>
<td>Ciprofloxacin*
(Cipro®)
Pregnancy: C; Lactation: Unsafe
Tabs: 250 mg, 500 mg, 750 mg - $$</td>
<td>Adolescent and Adult: 500 mg twice daily for 3 days.</td>
<td>Food: Take on empty stomach 1 hour before or 2 hours after a meal. May take with food if it causes GI upset, but avoid large amounts of dairy products. May take 2 hours before or 6 hours after sucralfate, antacids, aluminum, magnesium, calcium, zinc, iron, sucralfate, vitamins, or mineral supplements.
Important side effects: Photosensitivity, dizziness.
Reduce dose in renal disease (CrCl <50 mL/min).</td>
</tr>
<tr>
<td>Erythromycin base*
(E-Mycin®, Ery-Tabs®)
Generics available
Pregnancy: B; Lactation: Safe
Tabs: 250 mg, 500 mg - <$
Caps: 250 mg</td>
<td>Adolescent and Adult: 500 mg four times daily for 7 days.</td>
<td>Food: May take with or without meals. Take with food if causes GI upset.
Important side effects: GI upset, hepatitis, drug interactions.</td>
</tr>
</table>

(continued)

GENITOURINARY – STD, Chancroid (*H. ducreyi*)

Drug, Its Forms and Dosage Increments	Children and Adult Dosages and Instructions	Information and Important Side Effects
Ceftriaxone (IM) (Rocephin®) Pregnancy: B; Lactation: Unk **Vials:** 250 mg - $, 500 mg, 1,000 mg	**Adolescent and Adult:** 250 mg IM × 1 dose.	**Important side effects:** Pain at injection site.

GENITOURINARY – STD, Chlamydia (*Chlamydia trachomatis*)

General statement: Instruct patient to refer sex partner for evaluation and treatment. Patient and partner should abstain from intercourse until after completion of course of therapy (7 days after single-dose therapy).

Drug, Its Forms and Dosage Increments	Children and Adult Dosages and Instructions	Information and Important Side Effects
Azithromycin* (Zithromax®) Pregnancy: B; Lactation: Unk **Tabs:** 250 mg - $$ **Powder for Oral Suspension:** 1 g - $$	**Child ≥45 kg and Adult:** 1 g PO × 1 dose.	**Food:** 1-g powder packet for oral suspension and tablets may be taken without regard to food. **Important side effects:** Nausea, diarrhea, elevated LFTs.
Doxycycline* (Vibramycin®) Generics available Pregnancy: D; Lactation: Unsafe **Caps:** 50 mg, 100 mg - <$ **Tabs:** 100 mg - <$	**Child ≥8 years and Adult:** 100 mg PO twice daily × 7 days.	**Food:** May take with food if GI upset occurs. Take 1 hour before or 2 hours after antacids, iron, milk, or other dairy products. Take with full glass of water to prevent esophagitis. **Important side effects:** Photosensitivity, use sunscreen. Esophagitis. May discolor fingernails.

Erythromycin Base* **Alternative** (E-Mycin®, Ery-Tab®) Generics available Pregnancy: B; Lactation: + **Tabs:** 250 mg, 333 mg, 500 mg - <$ **Caps:** 250 mg - <$ *May be less effective than recommended alternatives. Reserve for Children <45 kg or others intolerant to recommended drugs.	**Children <45 kg:** 50 mg/kg/day (NTE 2000 mg/day) in divided doses four times daily for 10-14 days. **Adolescents and Adult:** 500 mg four times daily for 7 days.	**Food:** May take with or without meals. Take with food if causes GI upset. **Important side effects:** GI upset, hepatitis, drug interactions.
Ofloxacin* (Floxin®) Pregnancy: C; Lactation:Unk **Tabs:** 200 mg, 300 mg, 400 mg - $$$$	**Adult:** 300 mg PO twice daily for 7 days.	**Food:** Take on empty stomach. Do not take within 2 hours of antacids, magnesium, calcium, zinc, iron, aluminum, sucralfate, vitamins, or mineral supplements. **Important side effects:** Nausea, photosensitivity, dizziness. **Reduce dose in renal disease (CrCl <50 mL/min).**

GENITOURINARY – STD, Chlamydia, Pregnancy (*Chlamydia trachomatis*)

Azithromycin* (Zithromax®) Pregnancy: B; Lactation: Unk **Tabs:** 250 mg - $$ **Powder for Oral Suspension:** 1 g - $$	**Adolescents and Adult:** 1 g PO × 1 dose.	**Food:** 1 g powder packet for oral suspension and tablets may be taken without regard to food. **Important side effects:** Nausea, diarrhea, elevated LFTs.

(continued)

Drug, Its Forms and Dosage Increments	Children and Adult Dosages and Instructions	Information and Important Side Effects
Erythromycin Base* (E-Mycin®) Generics available Pregnancy: B; Lactation: Safe **Tabs:** 250 mg, 500 mg - <$ **Caps:** 250 mg - <$	**Adolescent and Adult:** 500 mg four times daily × 7 days (recommended) or, if gastrointestinal intolerance, 250 mg four times daily × 14 days. Not as effective as azithromycin. Consider retesting in 2-3 weeks.	**Food:** May take with or without meals. Take with food if causes GI upset. **Important side effects:** GI upset, hepatitis, drug interactions.

GENITOURINARY – STD, Gonorrhea, Uncomplicated Urethritis, Cervicitis, or Proctitis (*Neisseria gonorrhoeae*) **General statement:** After neonatal period, sexual abuse is most common cause of gonococcal infection in preadolescent children. Coinfection with *C. trachomatis* may be common; consider treating for dual infection.

Drug, Its Forms and Dosage Increments	Children and Adult Dosages and Instructions	Information and Important Side Effects
Ceftriaxone (IM) (Rocephin®) Pregnancy: B; Lactation: Unk **Vials:** 250 mg, 500 mg, 1,000 mg - $	**Children and Adult:** 125 mg IM × 1 dose. **Children ≥45 kg and Adults: Treat with concomitant azithromycin or doxycycline for presumptive *C. trachomatis*.**	**Important side effects:** Pain at injection site.
Cefixime (Suprax®) Pregnancy: B; Lactation: Unk **Tabs:** 200 mg, 400 mg - <$ **Oral Susp:** 100 mg/5 mL - $$$$	**Children:** 8 mg/kg (max 400 mg) × 1 dose. **>50 kg and Adult:** 400 mg × 1 dose. **Children ≥45 kg and Adults treat with concomitant azithromycin or doxycycline for presumptive *C. trachomatis*.**	**Food:** May administer on empty stomach. May administer with food to reduce GI distress. **Important side effects:** Nausea, diarrhea.
Ciprofloxacin* (Cipro®) Pregnancy: C; Lactation: Unsafe **Tabs:** 250 mg, 500 mg - <$	**≥18 years:** 500 mg × 1 dose. **Treat with concomitant azithromycin or doxycycline for presumptive *C. trachomatis*.**	**Food:** Take on empty stomach 1 hour before or 2 hours after a meal. May take with food if it causes GI upset, but avoid large amounts of dairy products. May take 2 hours before or 6 hours

		after sucralfate, antacids, aluminum, magnesium, calcium, zinc, iron, sucralfate, vitamins, or mineral supplements. **Important side effects:** Photosensitivity, dizziness.
Ofloxacin* (Floxin®) Pregnancy: C; Lactation: Unk **Tabs:** 200 mg, 300 mg, 400 mg - <$	**Adult:** 400 mg × 1 dose. **Treat with concomitant azithromycin or doxycycline for presumptive *C. trachomatis.***	**Food:** Take on empty stomach. Do not take within 2 hours of antacids, magnesium, calcium, zinc, iron, aluminum, sucralfate, vitamins, or mineral supplements. **Important side effects:** Nausea, photosensitivity, dizziness.
Azithromycin* (Zithromax®) Pregnancy: B; Lactation: Unk **Tabs:** 250 mg - $$ **Powder for Oral Suspension:** 1 g - $$	**Children ≥45 kg and Adult:** 1 g × 1 dose. **Use in conjunction with cefixime, ceftriaxone, ciprofloxacin, or ofloxacin.**	**Food:** 1-g powder packet for oral suspension and tablets may be taken without regard to food. **Important side effects:** Nausea, diarrhea, elevated LFTs.
Doxycycline* (Vibramycin®) Generics available Pregnancy: D; Lactation: Unsafe **Caps:** 50 mg, 100 mg - <$ **Tabs:** 100 mg - <$	**Children ≥8 years and Adult:** 100 mg PO twice daily for 7 days. **Use in conjunction with cefixime, ceftriaxone, ciprofloxacin, or ofloxacin.**	**Food:** May take with food if GI upset occurs. Take 1 hour before or 2 hours after antacids, iron, milk, or other dairy products. Take with full glass of water to prevent esophagitis. **Important side effects:** Photosensitivity, use sunscreen. Esophagitis. May discolor fingernails.

(continued)

Drug, Its Forms and Dosage Increments	Children and Adult Dosages and Instructions	Information and Important Side Effects
GENITOURINARY - STD, Gonorrhea, Pregnancy, Uncomplicated Urethritis, Cervicitis, or Proctitis (*Neisseria gonorrhoeae*)		
Ceftriaxone (IM) (Rocephin®) Pregnancy: B; Lactation: Unk **Vials:** 250 mg, 500 mg, 1,000 mg **Vials with 2.1 mL lidocaine for IM injection:** 500 mg, 1,000 mg	**Adolescent and Adults:** 125 mg IM × 1 dose. **Treat with concomitant erythromycin or amoxicillin for presumptive *C. trachomatis.***	**Important side effects:** Pain at injection site.
Spectinomycin* (IM) **Alternative for cephalosporin allergy.** (Trobicin®) Pregnancy: B; Lactation: Unk **IM Injection:** 2 g - $$	**Adolescents and Adult:** 2 g IM × 1 dose. **Treat with concomitant erythromycin for presumptive *C. trachomatis.***	
Amoxicillin (Amoxil®) Generics available Pregnancy: B; Lactation: Safe **Caps:** 250 mg, 500 mg - <$ **Tabs:** 500 mg, 875 mg - $	**Adolescents and Adult:** 500 mg three times daily for 7 days. **Use in conjunction with ceftriaxone, cefixime, or spectinomycin.**	**Food:** May be taken without regard to food. **Important side effects:** Diarrhea and nausea. May cause nonallergic maculopapular rash.
Cefixime (Suprax®) Pregnancy: B; Lactation: Unk **Tabs:** 200 mg, 400 mg - <$	**Adolescent and Adult:** 400 mg × 1 dose. **Treat with concomitant erythromycin or amoxicillin for presumptive *C. trachomatis.***	**Food:** May administer on empty stomach. May administer with food to reduce GI distress. **Important side effects:** Nausea, diarrhea.

Erythromycin Base*
(E-Mycin®)
Generics available
Pregnancy: B; Lactation: Unsafe
Tabs: 250 mg, 500 mg - <$
Caps: 250 mg - <$

Adolescents and Adult: 500 mg four times daily × 7 days (recommended) or if gastrointestinal intolerance 250 mg four times daily × 14 days.
Use in conjunction with ceftriaxone, cefixime, or spectinomycin.

Food: May take with or without meals. Take with food if causes GI upset.
Important side effects: GI upset, hepatitis, drug interactions.

GENITOURINARY – STD, Genital Herpes, First Episode (Herpes simplex virus) Not a cure but may reduce duration of outbreak.

Acyclovir*
(Zovirax®)
Pregnancy: C; Lactation: Safe
Caps: 200 mg - $
Tabs: 400 mg, 800 mg - $-$$
Oral Susp: 200 mg/5 mL - >$$$$

Children: 80 mg/kg/day (up to equivalent adult doses) in divided doses 3-5 times daily for 7-10 days.
200 mg/ 5 mL @ 80 mg/kg/day
10 kg (22 lb) = 6.7 mL Q8H
15 kg (33 lb) = 10 mL Q8H
≥15 kg = Use adult dose.
Adults: 400 mg three times daily for 7-10 days **or** 200 mg five times daily for 7-10 days.

Food: May be taken without regard to food. **Encourage fluids.**
Important side effects: Headache, dizziness, nausea, seizures, bone-marrow suppression, nephrotoxicity.
Reduce dose in renal disease (CrCl <10 mL/min).

Famciclovir*
(Famvir®)
Pregnancy: B; Lactation: Unsafe
Tabs: 125 mg, 250 mg, 500 mg - >$$$$

Adult: 250 mg PO three times daily for 7-10 days.

Food: May take without regard to food.
Important side effects: Nausea, headache, dizziness.
Reduce dose in renal disease (CrCl <40 mL/min).

Valacyclovir*
(Valtrex®)
Pregnancy: B; Lactation: Unk

Adult: 1,000 mg PO twice daily for 7-10 days.

Food: May take without regard to food.
Important side effects: Nausea, headache, dizziness

(continued)

Drug, Its Forms and Dosage Increments	Children and Adult Dosages and Instructions	Information and Important Side Effects
Tabs: 500 mg, 1,000 mg - $$$		**Reduce dose in renal disease (CrCl <30 mL/min).**

GENITOURINARY – STD, Genital Herpes, Recurrent (Herpes simplex virus)

Drug, Its Forms and Dosage Increments	Children and Adult Dosages and Instructions	Information and Important Side Effects
Acyclovir* (Zovirax®) Pregnancy: C; Lactation: Safe **Caps:** 200 mg - $ **Tabs:** 400 mg, 800 mg - $-$$ **Oral Susp:** 200 mg/5 mL - >$$$$	**Children:** 80 mg/kg/day (up to equivalent adult doses) in divided doses 2-5 times daily for 5 days. **200 mg/ 5 mL @ 80 mg/kg/day** 10 kg (22 lb) = 6.7 mL Q8H 15 kg (33 lb) = 10 mL Q8H ≥15 kg = Use adult dose. **Adults:** 400 mg three times daily for 5 days **or** 200 mg five times daily for 5 days **or** 800 mg twice daily for 5 days.	**Food:** May be taken without regard to food. Encourage fluids. **Important side effects:** Headache, dizziness, nausea, seizures, bone-marrow suppression, nephrotoxicity. **Reduce dose in renal disease (CrCl <10 mL/min).**
Famciclovir* (Famvir®) Pregnancy: B; Lactation: Unsafe **Tabs:** 125 mg, 250 mg, 500 mg - $$	**Adult:** 125 mg PO twice daily for 5 days.	**Food:** May take without regard to food. **Important side effects:** Nausea, headache, dizziness. **Reduce dose in renal disease (CrCl <40 mL/min).**
Valacyclovir* (Valtrex®) Pregnancy: B; Lactation: Unk **Tabs:** 500 mg, 1,000 mg - $$	**Adult:** 500 mg PO twice daily for 5 days.	**Food:** May take without regard to food. **Important side effects:** Nausea, headache, dizziness. **Reduce dose in renal disease (CrCl <30 mL/min).**

GENITOURINARY – STD, Genital Herpes, Suppressive Tx (Herpes simplex virus)

Drug	Dosage	Comments
Acyclovir* (Zovirax®) Pregnancy: C; Lactation: Safe **Caps:** 200 mg **Tabs:** 400 mg, 800 mg **Oral Susp:** 200 mg/5 mL	**Children:** 80 mg/kg/day (max 800-1,000 mg) in divided doses 2-5 times daily. **200 mg/ 5 mL @ 80 mg/kg/day** 5 kg (22 lb) = 5 mL Q12H ≥10 kg = 10 mL Q12H **Adults:** 400 mg PO twice daily.	**Food:** May be taken without regard to food. Encourage fluids. **Important side effects:** Headache, dizziness, nausea, seizures, bone-marrow suppression, nephrotoxicity. **Reduce dose in renal disease (CrCl <10 mL/min).**
Famciclovir* (Famvir®) Pregnancy: B; Lactation: Unsafe **Tabs:** 125 mg, 250 mg, 500 mg	**Adult:** 250 mg PO twice daily.	**Food:** May take without regard to food. **Important side effects:** Nausea, headache, dizziness. **Reduce dose in renal disease (CrCl <40 mL/min).**
Valacyclovir* (Valtrex®) Pregnancy: B; Lactation: Unk **Tabs:** 500 mg, 1,000 mg	**Adult:** 500-1,000 mg PO once daily.	**Food:** May take without regard to food. **Important side effects:** Nausea, headache, dizziness. **Reduce dose in renal disease (CrCl <30 mL/min).**

GENITOURINARY – STD, Genital Herpes, Pregnancy (Herpes simplex virus)

General statement: Use of acyclovir and valacyclovir in pregnancy are under investigation, but preliminary evidence has not found them to be detrimental to the fetus. Pregnant women who receive these drugs should be reported to the CDC/Glaxo SmithKline registry (800) 722-9292, extension 38465.

Drug	Dosage	Comments
Acyclovir* (Zovirax®) Pregnancy: C; Lactation: Safe	**Adults:** 400 mg three times daily for 7-10 days **or** 200 mg five times daily for 7-10 days.	**Food:** May be taken without regard to food. Encourage fluids.

(continued)

Drug, Its Forms and Dosage Increments	Children and Adult Dosages and Instructions	Information and Important Side Effects
Caps: 200 mg - $ **Tabs:** 400 mg, 800 mg - $		**Important side effects:** Headache, dizziness, nausea, seizures, bone-marrow suppression, nephrotoxicity. **Reduce dose in renal disease (CrCl <10 mL/min).**
Valacyclovir* (Valtrex®) Pregnancy: B; Lactation: Unk **Tabs:** 500 mg, 1,000 mg - $$$$	**Adult:** 1,000 mg twice daily for 7-10 days.	**Food:** May take without regard to food. **Important side effects:** Nausea, headache, dizziness. **Reduce dose in renal disease (CrCl <30 mL/min).**

GENITOURINARY – STD, Syphilis – Primary, Secondary, and Early Latent (*Treponema pallidum*)

General statement: Penicillin G is the preferred drug for treatment of syphilis. Pregnant patients and patients with neurosyphilis with a history of allergy to penicillin should be desensitized and treated with penicillin if possible.

Drug, Its Forms and Dosage Increments	Children and Adult Dosages and Instructions	Information and Important Side Effects
Penicillin G benzathine (Bicillin L-A®, Permapen®) Pregnancy: B; Lactation: Unk **Injection (IM only):** 300,000 U/mL and 600,000 U/mL (1 mL, 2 mL, 4 mL)	**Children:** 50,000 U/kg up to adult dose IM × 1 dose. **Adolescents and Adult:** 2.4 mU IM × 1, divided in two sites.	**Important side effects:** Jarisch-Herxheimer reaction, pain at injection site. **Caution:** Do not give IV, IA, or SC. Use with caution in persons with history of seizures.
Doxycycline* (Vibramycin®) Generics available Pregnancy: D; Lactation: Unsafe **Caps:** 50 mg, 100 mg - <$	**Adolescents and Adults:** 100 mg twice daily for 14 days.	**Food:** May take with food if GI upset occurs. Take 1 hour before or 2 hours after antacids, iron, milk, or other dairy

Drug	Dose	Comments
Tabs: 100 mg - <$ ***For use only in nonpregnant patients with documented penicillin allergy, likely good compliance and follow-up.**		products. Take with full glass of water to prevent esophagitis. **Important side effects:** Photosensitivity, use sunscreen. Esophagitis. May discolor fingernails.
Tetracycline* (Sumycin®, Achromycin V®) Generics available Pregnancy: D; Lactation: Unsafe **Caps:** 250 mg, 500 mg - <$ **Tabs:** 250 mg, 500 mg - <$ ***For use only in nonpregnant patients with documented penicillin allergy, likely good compliance and follow-up.**	**Adult:** 500 mg four times daily for 14 days.	**Food:** Take 1 hour before or 2 hours after meals. Do not take with dairy products, antacids, calcium, zinc, or iron products. Take with large glass of water to prevent esophagitis. **Important side effects:** GI upset, esophagitis, photosensitivity, discoloration of fingernails, superinfection (vaginal candidiasis). Use with caution in liver or renal disease.

GENITOURINARY – STD, Syphilis – Pregnancy (*Treponema pallidum*)

Drug	Dose	Comments
<u>Penicillin G benzathine</u> (Bicillin L-A®, Permapen®) Pregnancy: B; Lactation: Unk **Injection (IM only):** 300,000 U/mL and 600,000 U/mL (1 mL, 2 mL, 4 mL)	**Adolescent and Adults:** 2.4 mU IM $\times$ 1, divided in two sites.	**Important side effects:** Jarisch-Herxheimer reaction, pain at injection site. **Caution:** Do not give IV, IA, or SC. Use with caution in persons with history of seizures.

(continued)

Drug, Its Forms and Dosage Increments	Children and Adult Dosages and Instructions	Information and Important Side Effects
GENITOURINARY – STD, Trichomoniasis (Trichomonas vaginalis) **General statement:** Effective alternatives to metronidazole are not available in the United States. Consider desensitizing persons with metronidazole allergy. Sex partners should be treated. Patient and partner should avoid sex until therapy is completed and they are asymptomatic.		
Metronidazole* (Flagyl®) Generics available Pregnancy: B; Lactation: Unsafe **Tabs:** 250 mg, 500 mg - <$	**Adolescents and Adult:** 2 g × 1 dose **or** 500 mg twice daily for 7 days.	**Food:** Administer on empty stomach unless GI upset occurs, then with food. **Important side effects:** Dizziness, headache, confusion, seizures, nausea, metallic taste, insomnia, paresthesias. May cause Disulfiram-like reaction – avoid alcohol.
GENITOURINARY – STD, Trichomoniasis – Pregnancy (*Trichomonas vaginalis*)		
Metronidazole* (Flagyl®) Generics available Pregnancy: B; Lactation: Unsafe **Tabs:** 250 mg, 500 mg - <$ *Consider deferring treatment until after first trimester.	**Adolescents and Adult:** 2 g PO × 1 dose.	**Food:** Administer on empty stomach unless GI upset occurs, then with food. **Important side effects:** Dizziness, headache, confusion, seizures, nausea, metallic taste, insomnia, paresthesias. Avoid alcohol.

GENITOURINARY – STD, Urethritis, Nongonococcal

General statement: Confirm urethritis and rule out gonococcal or chlamydial infection. Patient should refer all sex partners within previous 60 days for evaluation and treatment.

Azithromycin* (Zithromax®) Pregnancy: B; Lactation: Unk **Tabs:** 250 mg - $$ **Powder for Oral Suspension:** 1 g - $$	**Adolescents and Adult:** 1 g × 1 dose.	**Food:** 1 g powder for oral suspension and tablet may be taken without regard to food. **Important side effects:** Nausea, diarrhea, elevated LFTs.
Doxycycline* (Vibramycin®) Generics available Pregnancy: D; Lactation: Unsafe **Caps:** 50 mg, 100 mg - <$ **Tabs:** 100 mg - <$	**Adolescents and Adults:** 100 mg twice daily for 7 days.	**Food:** May take with food if GI upset occurs. Take 1 hour before or 2 hours after antacids, iron, milk, or other dairy products. Take with full glass of water to prevent esophagitis. **Important side effects:** Photosensitivity, use sunscreen. Esophagitis. May discolor fingernails.
Erythromycin Base* **Alternative** (E-Mycin®) Generics available Pregnancy: B; Lactation: Safe **Tabs:** 250 mg, 500 mg - <$ **Caps:** 250 mg - <$	**Adolescents and Adults:** 500 mg four times daily × 7 days (recommended) or, if gastrointestinal intolerance, 250 mg four times daily × 14 days.	**Food:** May take with or without meals. Take with food if causes GI upset. **Important side effects:** GI upset, hepatitis, drug interactions.
Ofloxacin* **Alternative** (Floxin®)	**Adult:** 300 mg twice daily for 7 days.	**Food:** Take on empty stomach. Do not take within 2 hours of antacids, magnesium, calcium, zinc, iron,

(continued)

Drug, Its Forms and Dosage Increments	Children and Adult Dosages and Instructions	Information and Important Side Effects
Pregnancy: C; Lactation: Unk **Tabs:** 200 mg, 300 mg, 400 mg - $$$		aluminum, sucralfate, vitamins, or mineral supplements. **Important side effects:** Nausea, photosensitivity, dizziness. **Reduce dose in renal disease (CrCl <30 mL/min).**

GENITOURINARY - STD, Urethritis, Nongonococcal, Recurrent, or Persistent

Drug, Its Forms and Dosage Increments	Children and Adult Dosages and Instructions	Information and Important Side Effects
Metronidazole* (Flagyl®) Generics available Pregnancy: B; Lactation: Unsafe **Tabs:** 250 mg, 500 mg - <$ ***Use in conjunction with erythromycin.**	**Adolescents and Adult:** 2 g × 1 dose.	**Food:** Administer on empty stomach unless GI upset occurs, then with food. **Important side effects:** Dizziness, headache, confusion, seizures, nausea, metallic taste, insomnia, paresthesias. **Avoid alcohol.**
Erythromycin Base* (E-Mycin®) Generics available Pregnancy: B; Lactation: Safe **Tabs:** 250 mg, 500 mg - <$ **Caps:** 250 mg - <$ ***Use in conjunction with metronidazole.**	**Adolescents and Adults:** 500 mg four times daily × 7 days.	**Food:** May take with or without meals. Take with food if causes GI upset. **Important side effects:** GI upset, hepatitis, drug interactions.

List of Drugs

Drug	Typical Dosing
Acetic acid 2%* VoSol® otic Generics available Pregnancy: Unk; Lactation: Unk **Solution:** 15-mL bottle	**Children/Adult:** Saturate cotton wick and insert in ear. Apply 3-5 drops to wick every 4-6 hours × 24 hours. Remove wick, then instill 3-5 drops in affected ear(s) 3-4 times daily for as long as needed.
Acetic acid 2% + Hydrocortisone 1%* VoSol HC® Otic Pregnancy: Unk; Lactation: Unk **Solution:** 10-mL bottle	**Children/Adult:** Saturate cotton wick and insert in ear. Apply 3-5 drops to wick every 4-6 hours × 24 hours. Remove wick, then instill 3-5 drops in affected ear(s) 3-4 times daily for as long as needed.
Acyclovir Zovirax® Generics available Pregnancy: C; Lactation: Safe **Caps:** 200 mg **Tabs:** 400 mg 800 mg **Suspension:** 200 mg/5 mL	**Children ≥2 years:** <40 kg: 20 mg/kg (maximum of 800 mg/dose) PO 4 times daily for 5 days. ≥40 kg: 800 mg PO 4 times daily for 5 days. **Adults:** Range: 200 mg PO three times daily (chronic suppression of herpes simplex) to 800 mg PO five times daily (treatment of acute herpes zoster). **Food:** May take without regard to food. **Maintain good hydration.** **Important side effects:** Headache, nausea, rash. Crystallization in renal tubes and renal dysfunction—maintain good hydration. CNS changes include lethargy, confusion, hallucinations, seizures, agitation, and coma. **Reduce dose in renal disease:** Normal dose 200 mg 5x/day: For CrCl <10 mL/min use 200 mg 2x/day Normal dose 400 mg 2x/day: For CrCl <10 mL/min use 200 mg 2x/day

Drug	Typical Dosing
	Normal dose 800 mg 5x/day: For CrCl 10-25 mL/min use 800 mg 3x/day For CrCl <10 mL/min use 800 mg 2x/day
Amoxicillin Amoxil®, Trimox® Generics available Pregnancy: B; Lactation: Safe **Caps:** 250 mg 500 mg **Tabs:** 500 mg 875 mg **Chewable Tab:** 125 mg, 200 mg, 250 mg, 400 mg 250 mg **Oral Susp:** 50 mg/mL 125 mg/5 mL 250 mg/5 mL 200 mg/5 mL 400 mg/5 mL	**Neonates and infants ≤3 months:** 20-30 mg/kg/day in divided doses Q12H. **Children >3 months:** 25-50 mg/kg/day (max 2-3 g/day) in divided doses Q8H or Q12H. **250 mg/5 mL at 50 mg/kg/day** 10 kg (22 lb) = 1 tsp (5 mL) Q12H 15 kg (33 lb) = 1 tsp (5 mL) Q8H 20 kg (44 lb) = 2 tsp (10 mL) Q12H >25 kg = Use adult dose. **Adult:** 250-500 mg PO Q8H or 500-875 mg PO Q12H. **Food:** May take with or without meals. **Important side effects:** Nausea, vomiting, diarrhea, agitation, seizures, rash, bleeding abnormalities, decreased WBC count, drug fever, superinfection. **Caution:** May cause nonallergic maculopapular rash, especially in patients with viral infection, infectious mononucleosis, or acute lymphocytic leukemia. **Reduce dose in renal disease:** CrCl 10-30 mL/min administer every 12 hours CrCl <10 mL/min administer every 24 hours
Amoxicillin/clavulanate Augmentin® Pregnancy: B; Lactation: Unk **Q12H Formulations:**	**Dosing: Based on Amoxicillin Component** **Neonates and infants <3 months: 125 mg/5 mL suspension** 30 mg/kg/day in divided doses Q12H.

(continued)

Drug	Typical Dosing
Tabs:	**Children ≥3 months up to 40 kg: Oral Suspension or Chewable Tablet**
500 mg/125 mg	25-45 mg/kg/day in divided doses Q12H using a Q12H formulation.
875 mg/125 mg	20-40 mg/kg/day in divided doses Q8H using a Q8H formulation.
Chewable Tabs:	**Multidrug-resistant *S. pneumonia* otitis media:**
200 mg/28.5 mg	80-90 mg/kg/day in divided doses Q12H.
400 mg/57 mg	**Children ≥40 mg to Adult:**
Oral Susp:	250 mg PO Q8H or 500 mg PO Q12H.
200 mg/28.5 mg/5 mL	Severe or respiratory tract infection 500 mg PO Q8H or 875 mg PO Q12H.
400 mg/57 mg/5 mL	**Q12H using 200 mg/5 mL susp or 200-mg chewable tablet @ 45 mg/kg/day**
Q8H Formulations:	9 kg (20 lb) = 1 tsp (or tab) (5 mL) Q12H
Tabs:	13 kg (29 lb) = 1½ tsp (or tab) (7.5 mL) Q12H
250 mg/125 mg	18 kg (40 lb) = 2 tsp (or tabs) (10 mL) Q12H
500 mg/125 mg	**Q12H using 400 mg/5 mL susp or 400-mg chewable tablet @ 45 mg/kg/day**
Chewable Tabs:	18 kg (40 lb) = 1 tsp (or tab) (5 mL) Q12H
125 mg/31.25 mg	27 kg (59 lb) = 1½ tsp (or tab) (7.5 mL) Q12H
250 mg/62.5 mg	35 kg (77 lb) = 2 tsp (or tabs) (10 mL) Q12H
Oral Susp:	>40 kg = Use adult dose (max 875 mg Q12H)
125 mg/31.25 mg/5 mL	**Q8H using 125 mg/5 mL susp or 125-mg chewable tablet @ 40 mg/kg/day**
250 mg/62.5 mg/5 mL	9 kg (21 lb) = 1 tsp (or tabs) (5 mL) Q8H
Augmentin ES-600 powder for oral	14 kg (31 lb) = 1½ tsp (or tab) (7.5 mL) Q8H
suspension with increased ratio	19 kg (42 lb) = 2 tsp (or tabs) (10 mL) Q8H
amoxicillin to clavulanic acid for	**Q8H using 250 mg/5 mL susp or 250-mg chewable tablet @ 40 mg/kg/day**
treatment of pediatric patients with	19 kg (42 lb) = 1 tsp (or tabs) (5 mL) Q8H
recurrent or persistent acute otitis	28 kg (62 lb) = 1½ tsp (or tab) (7.5 mL) Q8H
media due to *S. pneumoniae*,	37 kg (81 lb) = 2 tsp (or tabs) (10 mL) Q8H
***H. influenzae*, or *M. catarrhalis*.**	**Q12H using 600 mg/5 mL ES-600 suspension for pediatric patients ≤ 40 kg with**
600 mg/42.9 mg/5 mL	**otitis media due to multi-drug resistant *S. pneumoniae***

Drug	Typical Dosing
	8 kg (18 lb) = 3 mL Q12H 12 kg (26 lb) = 4.5 mL Q12H 16 kg (35 lb) = 6 mL Q12H 20 kg (44 lb) = 7.5 mL Q12H 24 kg (53 lb) = 9 mL Q12H 28 kg (62 lb) = 10.5 mL Q12H 32 kg (70 lb) = 12 mL Q12H 36 kg (79 lb) = 13.5 mL Q12H **Food:** Advise taking with food. May administer with or without meals, however GI intolerance and diarrhea may be reduced if taken with meals. **Side effects:** Diarrhea (common), nausea, vomiting, rash, agitation, seizures, bleeding abnormalities, decreased WBC count, drug fever, superinfection. **Caution:** May cause nonallergic maculopapular rash, especially in patients with viral infection, mononucleosis, or acute lymphocytic leukemia. **Use with caution in hepatic disease.** **Reduce dose in renal disease:** CrCl 10-30 mL/min use a Q8H formulation Q12H CrCl <10 mL/min use a Q8H formulation Q24H **Note:** Q8H and Q12H formulations are not interchangeable due to different ratio of clavulanic acid. Two 250 mg/125 mg tablets are not equivalent to one 500 mg/125 mg tablet. 250 mg tablet is not equivalent to 250-mg chewable tablet. 200-mg and 400-mg suspensions and tablets contain phenylalanine and should be avoided in phenylketonurics.
Ampicillin Principen®, Omnipen®	**Children:** 50-100 mg/kg/day (max 2-3 g/day) in divided doses Q6H. **Adults:** 250-500 mg PO Q6H.

(continued)

Drug	Typical Dosing
Generics available Pregnancy: B; Lactation: Unknown **Caps:** 250 mg 500 mg **Oral Susp:** 125 mg/5 mL 250 mg/5 mL	**Food:** Administer on an empty stomach 1-2 hours before food. **Important side effects:** Nausea, vomiting, diarrhea, agitation, seizures, rash, bleeding abnormalities, decreased WBC count, drug fever, superinfection. **Caution:** May cause nonallergic maculopapular rash (5-10% of children), especially in patients with viral infection, infectious mononucleosis, or acute lymphocytic leukemia. **Reduce dose in renal disease:** CrCl 10-30 mL/min administer every 8-12 hours. CrCl <10 mL/min administer every 12 hours. **Ampicillin has comparable coverage to amoxicillin; however, amoxicillin has improved oral absorption and requires less frequent dosing.**
Azithromycin* Zithromax® Pregnancy: B; Lactation: Unk **Tabs:** 250 mg 600 mg Z-Pak = 250 mg tabs with instructions to take 500 mg on day 1 and 250 mg Q24H on days 2-5. **Oral Susp:** 100 mg/5 mL 200 mg/5 mL 1-g packet	**Children**: **Acute otitis media/community-acquired pneumonia in children ≥6 months:** 10 mg/kg (NTE 500 mg) once on the first day, followed by 5 mg/kg/day (NTE 250 mg) on days 2-5. **Pharyngitis/tonsillitis in children ≥2 years:** 12 mg/kg/day (NTE 500 mg) daily for 5 days. **Adult: Dispense Z-Pak.** Review specific disease states for dosing in sexually transmitted diseases and MAC. **Food:** Oral suspension should be taken 1 hour before or 2 hours after food. Tablets may be taken without regard to food. **Important side effects:** Nausea, diarrhea, elevated LFTs. **Caution**: Significant drug interactions may occur with pimozide (avoid), cyclosporine, HMG-CoA reductase inhibitors. Use with caution in hepatic disease.
Cefaclor Ceclor®	**Children ≥1 month:** **Usual dose:** 20 mg/kg/day (max 1,000 mg/day) in divided doses every 8 hours.

Drug	Typical Dosing
Pregnancy: B; Lactation: Unk **Caps:** 250 mg 500 mg **Tabs, Extended Release (CD):** 375 mg 500 mg **Powder for Oral Suspension:** 125 mg/5 mL 187 mg/5 mL 250 mg/5 mL 375 mg/5 mL	**Severe or Otitis Media:** 40 mg/kg/day (max 1,000 mg/day) in divided doses every 8 or 12 hours. **125 mg/5 mL @ 20 mg/kg/day (double for 40 mg/kg/day)** 9 kg (20 lb) = ½ tsp (2.5 mL) Q8H 18 kg (40 lb) = 1 tsp (5 mL) Q8H **250 mg/5 mL @ 20 mg/kg/day (double for 40 mg/kg/day)** 18 kg (40 lb) = ½ tsp (2.5 mL) Q8H 27 kg (50 lb) = ¾ tsp Q8H 36 kg (80 lb) = 1 tsp (5 mL) Q8H **Child ≥36 kg and Adult:** Capsules: 250-500 mg PO every 8 hours Extended release tablets: 375-500 mg PO every 12 hours **Food:** Capsules and oral suspension may be taken without regard to food. May take with food to reduce GI upset. Tablets should be taken with food. **Important side effects:** Nausea, vomiting, diarrhea, rash, elevated LFTs. **Caution:** Avoid use in patients with history of severe penicillin allergy. Use with caution in patients with history of seizures. **Reduce dose in severe renal disease:** CrCl <10 mL/min administer 50% of the usual dose.
Cefadroxil Duricef® Generics available Pregnancy: B; Lactation: Unknown **Caps:** 500 mg **Tabs:** 1 g	**Children:** 30 mg/kg/day (max 2000 mg/day) PO in divided doses once or twice daily (depends upon indication). **250 mg/5 mL @ 30 mg/kg/day** 9 kg (20 lb) = ½ tsp (2.5 mL) Q12H or 1 tsp (5 mL) Q24H 18 kg (40 lb) = 1 tsp (5 mL) Q12H or 2 tsp (10 mL) Q24H 27 kg (60 lb) = 2 tsp (10 mL) Q12H or 4 tsp (20 mL) Q24H

(continued)

Drug	Typical Dosing
Powder for Oral Suspension: 125 mg/5 mL 250 mg/5 mL 500 mg/5 mL	**Adult:** 1,000-2000 mg/day PO in divided doses once or twice daily. **Food:** May be taken without regard to food. May take with food to reduce GI upset. **Important side effects:** Nausea, vomiting, rash, diarrhea, elevated LFTs. **Caution:** Avoid use in patients with history of severe penicillin allergy. Use with caution in patients with history of seizures. **Reduce dose in renal disease:** CrCl 10-25 mL/min increase dose interval to every 24 hours. CrCl <10 mL/min increase dose interval to every 36 hours.
Cefdinir Omnicef® Pregnancy: B; Lactation: Unk **Caps:** 300 mg **Oral Susp:** 125 mg/5 mL	**Children ≥6 months to 12 years:** 14 mg/kg/day PO in one or two divided doses (depends on indication). **≥13 years to Adult:** 300 mg PO two times daily or 600 mg once daily (depends on indication). **125 mg/5 mL** 9 kg (20 lb) = ½ tsp (2.5 mL) Q12H or 1 tsp (5 mL) daily 18 kg (40 lb) = 1 tsp (5 mL) Q12H or 2 tsp (10 mL) daily 27 kg (60 lb) = 1½ tsp (7.5 mL) Q12H or 1 tbsp (15 mL) daily **Food:** May be taken without regard to food. May take with food to reduce GI upset. **Important side effects:** Nausea, vomiting, rash, diarrhea, elevated LFTs. **Caution:** Avoid use in patients with history of severe penicillin allergy. Use with caution in patients with history of seizures. **Reduce dose in renal disease:** CrCl <30 mL/min use 300 mg once daily.
Cefixime Suprax® Pregnancy: B; Lactation: Unk	**Children ≥6 months and <12 years or <50 kg:** 8 mg/kg/day PO once daily or 4 mg/kg/day PO two times daily (max 400 mg/day). **100 mg/5 mL** 12.5 kg (27.5 lb) = ½ tsp (2.5 mL) Q12H or 1 tsp (5 mL) daily

Drug	Typical Dosing
Tabs: 200 mg 400 mg **Powder for Oral Suspension:** 100 mg/5 mL	19 kg (42 lb) = ¾ tsp Q12H or 1½ tsp (7.5 mL) daily 25 kg (55 lb) = 1 tsp (5 mL) Q12H or 2 tsp (10 mL) daily 38 kg (77 lb) = 1½ (7.5 mL) Q12H or 1 tbsp (15 mL) daily >50 kg (110 lb) = Use adult dose. **Children ≥50 kg or ≥12 years to Adult:** 400 mg PO once daily or 200 mg PO twice daily. **Food:** May be taken without regard to food. May take with food to reduce GI upset. **Important side effects:** Nausea, vomiting, rash, diarrhea, elevated LFTs. **Caution:** Avoid use in patients with history of severe penicillin allergy. Use with caution in patients with history of seizures. **Reduce dose in renal disease:** CrCl 21-60 mL/min administer 75% of usual dose. CrCl <20 mL/min administer 50% of usual dose.
Cefpodoxime Vantin® Pregnancy: B; Lactation: Unk **Tabs:** 100 mg 200 mg **Granules for Oral Suspension:** 50 mg/5 mL 100 mg/5 mL	**Children ≥5 months to 12 years:** 10 mg/kg/day in one or two divided doses (max 400 mg/day). **50 mg/5 mL @ 10 mg/kg/day** 10 kg (22 lb) = 1 tsp (5 mL) Q12H or 2 tsp (10 mL) daily 15 kg (33 lb) = 1½ tsp (7.5 mL) Q12H or 3 tsp (15 mL) daily **100 mg/5 mL @10 mg/kg/day** 15 kg (33 lb) = ¾ tsp Q12H or 1½ tsp (7.5 mL) daily 20 kg (44 lb) = 1 tsp (5 mL) Q12H 30 kg (66 lb) = 1½ tsp (7.5 mL) Q12H or 3 tsp (15 mL) daily 40 kg (88 lb) = Use adult dose. **≥12 years to Adult:** 100-400 mg two times daily. **Food:** Take tablet with food. Suspension may be taken without regard to food.

(continued)

Drug	Typical Dosing
	Important side effects: Nausea, vomiting, rash, diarrhea, elevated LFTs. **Caution:** Avoid use in patients with history of severe penicillin allergy. Use with caution in patients with history of seizures. **Reduce dose in renal disease.** CrCl <30 mL/min decrease dosing interval to once daily.
Cefprozil Cefzil® Pregnancy: B; Lactation: Unk **Tabs:** 250 mg 500 mg **Powder for Oral Suspension:** 125 mg/5 mL 250 mg/5 mL	**Children ≥6 months to 12 years:** 7.5-15 mg/kg/day in divided doses 2 times daily (max 1,000 mg/day). **250 mg/5 mL @ 30 mg/kg/day** 9.1 kg (20 lb) = ½ tsp (2.5 mL) Q12H 13.6 kg (30 lb) = ¾ tsp Q12H 18.2 kg (40 lb) = 1 tsp (5 mL) Q12H 27 kg (60 lb) = 1½ tsp (7.5 mL) Q12H 31 kg (70 lb) = Use adult dose. **≥13 years to Adult:** 250 mg Q12H or 500 mg once or twice daily. **Food:** May be taken without regard to food. May take with food to reduce GI upset. **Important side effects:** Nausea, vomiting, rash, diarrhea, elevated LFTs. **Caution:** Avoid use in patients with history of severe penicillin allergy. Use with caution in patients with history of seizures. **Reduce dose in renal disease:** CrCl <30 mL/min administer 50% of usual dose at standard dosing interval.
Ceftriaxone Rocephin® Pregnancy: B; Lactation: Unk **Powder for IM or IV injection:** 250 mg, 500 mg, 1,000 mg	**Children:** 25-75 mg/kg/day IM or IV in one or two divided doses (max 2000 mg/day) **Adult:** Usual dose 250 mg-2 g IM or IV once daily. Maximum dose 2 g Q12H. **Important side effects:** Rash, diarrhea, elevated LFTs. **Reduce dose in patients with combined liver disease and significant renal disease.**

Drug	Typical Dosing
	Caution: Avoid use in patients with history of severe penicillin allergy. Use with caution in patients with history of seizures. Use with caution in patients with history of biliary disease.
Cefuroxime axetil Ceftin® Pregnancy: B; Lactation: Unsafe **Tabs:** 125 mg 250 mg 500 mg **Powder for Oral Suspension:** 125 mg/5 mL 250 mg/5 mL **Note:** Tablets and oral suspension are not considered bioequivalent and cannot be directly substituted on a mg/mg basis.	**Children ≥3 months to 12 years:** 20-30 mg/kg/day in divided doses 2 times daily (maximum 1,000 mg/day). **125 mg/5 mL @ 20 mg/kg/day** 6 kg (13 lb) = ½ tsp (2.5 mL) Q12H 12 kg (26 lb) = 1 tsp (5 mL) Q12H 18 kg (40 lb) = 1½ tsp (7.5 mL) Q12H **125 mg/5 mL @ 30 mg/kg/day** 8 kg (18 lb) = 1 tsp (5 mL) Q12H 12.5 kg (27 lb) = 1½ tsp (7.5 mL) Q12H 17 kg (37 lb) = 2 tsp (10 mL) Q12H 25 kg (55 lb) = 1 tbsp (15 mL) Q12H 33 kg (73 lb) = Use adult dose. **250 mg/5 mL @ 30 mg/kg/day** 8 kg (18 lb) = ½ tsp (2.5 mL) Q12H 16 kg (36 lb) = 1 tsp (5 mL) Q12H 24 kg (54 lb) = 1½ tsp (7.5 mL) Q12H **≥13 years to Adult:** 250-500 mg Q12H. **Food:** Suspension should be taken with food. Tablets may be taken without regard to food. May administer with food to reduce GI upset. **Important side effects:** Nausea, vomiting, rash, diarrhea, elevated LFTs. **Caution:** Avoid use in patients with history of severe penicillin allergy. Use with caution in patients with history of seizures.

(continued)

Drug	Typical Dosing
	Reduce dose in renal disease: CrCl 10-29 mL/min give standard dose every 24 hours CrCl <10 mL/min give standard dose every 48 hours
Cephalexin Keflex® Generics available Pregnancy: B; Lactation: Unk **Caps:** 250 mg 500 mg **Tabs:** 250 mg 500 mg 1 g **Powder for Oral Suspension:** 125 mg/5 mL 250 mg/5 mL	**Children:** Usual dose 25-50 mg/kg/day in divided doses 2 to 4 times daily (max 4 g/day). **125 mg/5 mL @ 25 mg/kg/day (double for 50 mg/kg/day)** 10 kg (22 lb) = 1 tsp (5 mL) Q12H 15 kg (33 lb) = 1 tsp (5 mL) Q8H **250 mg/5 mL @ 25 mg/kg/day (double for 50 mg/kg/day)** 20 kg (44 lb) = 1 tsp (5 mL) Q12H or ½ tsp (2.5 mL) Q6H 40 kg (88 lb) = 1 tsp (5 mL) Q6H >40 kg = Use adult dose. **Adult:** 1-4 g daily in 2 to 4 divided doses. **Food:** May take with food if GI upset occurs. **Important side effects:** Nausea, vomiting, rash, diarrhea, elevated LFTs. **Caution:** Avoid use in patients with history of severe penicillin allergy. Use with caution in patients with history of seizures. **Reduce dose in renal disease:** CrCl 10-40 mL/min give standard dose every 8-12 hours CrCl <10 mL/min give standard dose every 12-24 hours
Ciprofloxacin* Cipro® Pregnancy: C; Lactation: Unsafe **Tabs:** 250 mg 500 mg 750 mg	**≥18 years to Adult:** 250-750 mg PO two times daily. **Food:** Take on empty stomach 1 hour before or 2 hours after a meal. Take 2 hours before or 6 hours after sucralfate, antacids, aluminum, magnesium, calcium, zinc, iron, sucralfate, vitamins, or mineral supplements. **Important side effects:** Photosensitivity, dizziness, headache, insomnia, rash (may be severe), seizures, superinfection, angina, atrial flutter, bronchospasm.

Drug	Typical Dosing
Oral Suspension: 250 mg/5 mL 500 mg/5 mL	**Drug Interactions:** May be significant with ciprofloxacin, especially caffeine, phenytoin, cyclosporine, warfarin, theophylline. **Reduce dose in renal disease:** CrCl 30-50 mL/min 250-500 mg PO Q12H CrCl 5-29 mL/min 250-500 mg PO Q18H
Clarithromycin* Biaxin® Pregnancy: C; Lactation: Unk **Tabs:** 250 mg 500 mg **Tabs, extended release (XL):** 500 mg **Granules for Oral Suspension:** 125 mg/5 mL 187.5 mg/5 mL 250 mg/5 mL	**Children ≥6 months:** 15 mg/kg/day (max 1,000 mg/day) in divided doses two times daily. **125 mg/5 mL** 9 kg (20 lb) = ½ tsp (2.5 mL) Q12H 17 kg (37 lb) = 1 tsp (5 mL) Q12H **250 mg/5 mL** 17 kg (37 lb) = ½ tsp (2.5 mL) Q12H 25 kg (55 lb) = ¾ tsp Q12H 33 kg (73 lb) = 1 tsp (5 mL) Q12H **Adult:** Usual dose 250-500 mg PO Q12H or extended release 1,000 mg PO once daily. Doses of 500 mg Q8H (*H. pylori* regimens) and 1,000 mg Q12H (atypical mycobacterial infections) have been used. **Food:** May be taken without regard to food. **Important side effects:** Diarrhea, nausea, vomiting, headache, taste disturbance, elevated BUN, elevated LFTs, abdominal pain, superinfection, rash, hearing loss. **Caution:** Drug interactions may be significant, especially: Fluconazole, pimozide (avoid), rifampin, warfarin, benzodiazepines, buspirone, carbamazepine, digoxin, cyclosporine, ergots, disopyramide, tacrolimus, HMG-CoA reductase inhibitors, theophylline, zidovudine, others. **Use with caution in persons with liver disease.**

(continued)

Drug	Typical Dosing
	Reduce dose in renal disease: CrCl <30 mL/min reduce dose by 50% or double dosing interval.
Clindamycin* Cleocin® Generics available Pregnancy: B; Lactation: Safe **Caps:** 75 mg 150 mg 300 mg **Granules for Oral Solution:** 75 mg/5 mL	**Children:** **Mild to moderate infection:** 10-15 mg/kg/day (max 1.8 g/day) PO in divided doses three or four times daily. **Severe infection:** 16-30 mg/kg/day (max 1.8 g/day) in divided doses three or four times daily. **75 mg/5 mL @ 10 mg/kg/day divided Q8H** 11 kg (25 lb) = ½ tsp (2.5 mL) Q8H 22 kg (50 lb) = 1 tsp (5 mL) Q8H 34 kg (74 lb) = 1½ tsp (7.5 mL) Q8H 45 kg (100 lb) = 2 tsp (10 mL) Q8H >45 kg = Use adult dose. **Adult:** **Mild to moderate infection:** 150-300 mg PO three to four times daily. **Severe infection:** 450 mg PO four times daily. **Food:** May take with or without meals. Take with full glass of water to prevent esophagitis. **Important side effects:** Diarrhea, may be severe. Nausea, vomiting, stomatitis, rash, jaundice, elevated LFTs, superinfection. **May cause severe, potentially fatal, colitis.** Encourage patient to report severe, persistent, or bloody diarrhea, abdominal cramping, or blood or mucus in stool. **Reduce dose in severe renal or hepatic disease.**
Clindamycin Topical* Cleocin T® Generics available	**Children:** Should not be needed until adolescence.

Drug	Typical Dosing
Pregnancy: B; Lactation: Safe **Gel 1%:** 30 g **Sol 1%:** 30 mL **Lotion 1%:** 60 mL	**Adolescent and Adult:** Apply two times daily after cleansing. May see improvement in 2-6 weeks; however, may require 12 weeks for full response. Continue as long as satisfactory response is maintained and significant side effects do not occur. **Important side effects:** Local irritation and dryness. May rarely cause diarrhea. **May cause severe, potentially fatal, colitis.** Encourage patient to report severe, persistent, or bloody diarrhea, abdominal cramping, or blood or mucus in stool. **Avoid contact with eye(s) and mucous membranes.**
Clotrimazole* Mycelex®, Lotrimin®, Gyne-Lotrimin®, Fungoid® Pregnancy: C (troche) B (others); Lactation: Unk **Troche:** 10 mg **Vaginal tablet (OTC):** 100 mg (7's) 200 mg (3's) 500 mg (1's) **Vaginal cream 1% (OTC):** 45 g with applicator **Topical cream 1%:** 15 g, 30 g, 45 g **Topical solution 1%:** 10, 30 mL **Topical lotion 1%:** 20, 30 mL	<u>Oral Troche</u> **Children ≥ 3 years and Adults:** Dissolve one troche in mouth slowly (15-30 minutes) 5 times daily for 7-10 days or until 2-3 days after symptoms cleared. **Important side effects:** Nausea, unpleasant sensation in mouth, elevated LFTs. **Use with caution in liver disease.** <u>Vaginal Products</u> **Adolescents and Adult - vaginal tablet:** 100 mg tablet intravaginally at bedtime × 7 days **or** 200 mg tablet intravaginally at bedtime × 3 days **or** 500 mg tablet intravaginally at bedtime once. **Adolescent and Adult - vaginal cream:** One applicator intravaginally at bedtime × 7 days. Remain lying down for 30 minutes after application. Avoid intercourse during therapy. Do not use tampons until therapy is complete. Cream or vaginal tablets may weaken latex condoms and diaphragms. **Important side effects:** Rash, burning, irritation, cramping. <u>Topical Products</u> Gently massage into affected area two times daily after washing and drying. Relief of pruritus usually occurs within 1 week. If no clinical improvement after 4 weeks, reevaluate.

(continued)

Drug	Typical Dosing
	Important side effects: Local irritation. **Caution:** Avoid contact with eye(s).
Cortisporin® Otic* Hydrocortisone 1% + polymyxin + neomycin Generics available Pregnancy: C; Lactation: Unk **Otic Solution and Suspension 1%**	**Children and Adult:** Instill 3-4 drops in affected ear(s) three or four times daily for 5-10 days. **Use suspension only for perforated TM.** **Important side effects:** Neomycin is sensitizing in some patients.
Dicloxacillin Dynapen®, Dycill® Generics available Pregnancy: B; Lactation: Unk **Caps:** 250 mg 500 mg **Powder for Oral Suspension:** 62.5 mg/5 mL	**Children <40 kg:** 12.5-50 mg/kg/day in divided doses four times daily (max 2 g/day) **62.5 mg/kg/day @ 25 mg/kg/day** 5 kg (11 lb) = ½ tsp (2.5 mL) Q6H 10 kg (22 lb) = 1 tsp (5 mL) Q6H 15 kg (33 lb) = 1½ tsp (7.5 mL) Q6H 20 kg (44 lb) = 2 tsp (10 mL) Q6H 30 kg (66 lb) = 3 tsp (15 mL) Q6H **Children ≥40 kg to Adult:** 125-500 mg PO every 6 hours. **Food:** Take 1 hour before or 2 hours after meals. **Important side effects:** Bad taste, GI upset, vomiting, diarrhea, agitation, seizures, rash, bleeding abnormalities, decreased WBC count, drug fever, superinfection. **Caution:** Avoid use in patients with history of severe penicillin allergy. Use with caution in patients with history of seizures. **Do not need to adjust dose in renal disease.**
Doxycycline* Vibramycin® Generics available Pregnancy: D; Lactation: Unsafe	**Children:** 2-4 mg/kg/day (max 200 mg/day) in two divided doses. **Children ≥8 years and Adult:** 50-100 mg twice daily. Use in children <8 years old is generally not advised because tetracyclines can retard skeletal development and stain dental enamel. Doxycycline may have a role in some

Drug	Typical Dosing
Caps: 50 mg 100 mg **Tabs:** 100 mg **Powder for Oral Suspension:** 25 mg/5 mL **Syrup:** 50 mg/5 mL	children <8 years old in certain tick-borne diseases. The dental risk is less than other tetracyclines and is related to duration of use. **Food:** May take with food if GI upset occurs. Take 1 hour before or 2 hours after antacids, iron, milk, or other dairy products. Take with full glass of water to minimize esophagitis. **Important side effects:** Photosensitivity, use sunscreen. Esophagitis, take with full glass of water. May discolor fingernails. Rash, nausea, diarrhea, superinfection, hepatitis. **Outdated tetracyclines are toxic and should not be used.**
Erythromycin base* E-Mycin®, Ery-Tab® Generics available Pregnancy: B; Lactation: Safe **Tabs:** 250 mg 333 mg 500 mg **Caps:** 250 mg Erythromycin base tablets and capsules are coated or delayed release to minimize GI irritation. They should not be chewed or crushed.	**Children**: 30-50 mg/kg/day in divided doses every 6 to 8 hours (max 2,000 mg/day). **Adult:** 250-500 mg every 6 to 12 hours or 333 mg PO every 8 hours. **Food:** Take 1 hour before or 2 hours after meals. If GI upset occurs may take with food. **Important side effects:** Diarrhea, nausea, vomiting, headache, abdominal pain, dizziness, elevated LFTs, superinfection, rash, hearing loss, cardiac arrhythmias. Advise patient to contact provider if prodromal signs of liver dysfunction occur, i.e., abdominal pain, yellowing of skin or eye(s), unusual tiredness, dark urine, or pale stools. **Caution:** Drug interactions may be significant, especially pimozide (avoid), alfentanil, bromocriptine, felodipine, sparfloxacin (avoid), grepafloxacin, methylprednisolone, rifampin, warfarin, benzodiazepines, buspirone, carbamazepine, digoxin, cyclosporine, ergots, disopyramide, tacrolimus, HMG-CoA reductase inhibitors, theophylline, zidovudine, cisapride, others. **Use with caution in persons with liver disease.**
Erythromycin Estolate Ilosone® Generics available Pregnancy: B; Lactation: Safe	**Children:** 30-50 mg/kg/day in divided doses every 6 to 12 hours (max 2,000 mg/day). **30 mg/kg/day with 125 mg/5 mL** 4 kg (9 lb) = ½ tsp (2.5 mL) Q12H 6 kg (14 lb) = ½ tsp (2.5 mL) Q8H

(continued)

Drug	Typical Dosing
Tabs: 500 mg **Caps:** 250 mg **Oral Suspension:** 125 mg/5 mL 250 mg/5 mL	8 kg (18 lb) = ½ tsp (2.5 mL) Q6H or 1 tsp (5 mL) Q12H 12 kg (27 lb) = 1 tsp (5 mL) Q8H 17 kg (36 lb) = 1 tsp (5 mL) Q6H or 2 tsp (10 mL) Q12H **30 mg/kg/day with 250 mg/5 mL** 12 kg (27 lb) = ½ tsp (2.5 mL) Q8H 17 kg (36 lb) = ½ tsp (2.5 mL) Q6H or 1 tsp (5 mL) Q12H 25 kg (55 lb) = 1 tsp (5 mL) Q8H 33 kg (73 lb) = 1 tsp (5 mL) Q6H or 2 tsp (10 mL) Q12H **Adult:** 250-500 mg PO every 6 to 12 hours. **Food:** Take 1 hour before or 2 hours after meals. If GI upset occurs may take with food. **Important side effects:** Diarrhea, nausea, vomiting, headache, abdominal pain, dizziness, elevated LFTs, superinfection, rash, hearing loss, cardiac arrhythmias. Advise patient to contact provider if prodromal signs of liver dysfunction occur, i.e., abdominal pain, yellowing of skin or eye(s), unusual tiredness, dark urine, or pale stools. **Caution:** Drug interactions may be significant, especially pimozide (avoid), alfentanil, bromocriptine, felodipine, sparfloxacin (avoid), grepafloxacin, methylprednisolone, rifampin, warfarin, benzodiazepines, buspirone, carbamazepine, digoxin, cyclosporine, ergots, disopyramide, tacrolimus, HMG-CoA reductase inhibitors, theophylline, zidovudine, cisapride, others. **Use with caution in persons with liver disease.**
Erythromycin ethylsuccinate* ESS®, EryPed® Generics available Pregnancy: B; Lactation: +	**Neonates:** ≤7 days: 20 mg/kg/day in divided doses every 12 hours >7 days, <1,200 g: 20 mg/kg/day in divided doses every 12 hours >7 days, 1,200-2,000 g: 30 mg/kg/day in divided doses every 8 hours

Drug	Typical Dosing
Tabs: 400 mg **Chewable Tabs:** 200 mg **Oral Suspension:** 200 mg/5 mL 400 mg/5 mL **Note:** Due to differences in absorption, 200 mg erythromycin ethylsuccinate is approximately equivalent to 125 mg or erythromycin base or estolate.	>7 days, >2,000 g: 30-40 mg/kg/day in divided doses every 6-12 hours **Infants and Children:** 30-50 mg/kg/day in divided doses every 6 to 8 hours (max 3.2 g/day) **30 mg/kg/day with 200 mg/5 mL** 5 kg (11 lb) = ¼ tsp Q8H 7 kg (15 lb) = ¼ tsp Q6H 10 kg (22 lb) = ½ tsp (2.5 mL) Q8H 14 kg (30 lb) = ½ tsp (2.5 mL) Q6H 20 kg (44 lb) = 1 tsp (5 mL) Q8H **Adults:** 400-800 mg PO every 6 to 12 hours. **Food:** Take 1 hour before or 2 hours after meals. If GI upset occurs may take with food. **Important side effects:** Diarrhea, nausea, vomiting, headache, abdominal pain, dizziness, elevated LFTs, superinfection, rash, hearing loss, cardiac arrhythmias. Advise patient to contact provider if prodromal signs of liver dysfunction occur, i.e., abdominal pain, yellowing of skin or eye(s), unusual tiredness, dark urine, or pale stools. **Caution:** Drug interactions may be significant, especially pimozide (avoid), alfentanil, bromocriptine, felodipine, sparfloxacin (avoid), grepafloxacin, methylprednisolone, rifampin, warfarin, benzodiazepines, buspirone, carbamazepine, digoxin, cyclosporine, ergots, disopyramide, tacrolimus, HMG-CoA reductase inhibitors, theophylline, zidovudine, cisapride, others. **Use with caution in persons with liver disease.**
Erythromycin and Sulfisoxazole Pediazole®, Eryzole® Generics available	**Children ≥2 months:** Dosing based on erythromycin component: 40-50 mg/kg/day (erythromycin) in divided doses every 6 to 8 hours (max 2 g erythromycin/day).

(continued)

Drug	Typical Dosing
Pregnancy: C; Lactation: Unknown **Oral Suspension:** Erythromycin ethylsuccinate 200 mg and sulfisoxazole 600 mg/5 mL	**Erythromycin 200 mg/sulfisoxazole 200 mg/5 mL** 6 kg (13 lb) = ½ tsp (2.5 mL) Q8H 8 kg (18 lb) = ½ tsp (2.5 mL) Q6H 16 kg (35 lb) = 1 tsp (5 mL) Q6H 24 kg (53 lb) = 1½ tsp (7.5 mL) Q6H ≥32 kg (70 lb) = 2 tsp (10 mL) Q6H **Adults:** Erythromycin 400 mg and sulfisoxazole 1200 mg PO every 6 hours. **Food:** May be taken with or without meals. Take with food if GI upset occurs. Maintain good hydration. **Important side effects:** Diarrhea, nausea, vomiting, headache, abdominal pain, photosensitivity, dizziness, elevated LFTs, superinfection, rash, hearing loss, cardiac arrhythmias. Advise patient to contact provider if prodromal signs of liver dysfunction occur, i.e., abdominal pain, yellowing of skin or eye(s), unusual tiredness, dark urine, or pale stools. **Caution:** Drug interactions may be significant, especially pimozide (avoid), alfentanil, bromocriptine, felodipine, sparfloxacin (avoid), grepafloxacin, methylprednisolone, rifampin, warfarin, benzodiazepines, buspirone, carbamazepine, digoxin, cyclosporine, ergots, disopyramide, tacrolimus, HMG-CoA reductase inhibitors, theophylline, zidovudine, cisapride, others. **Use with caution in persons with liver disease, G-6-PD deficiency.**
Erythromycin Topical* Erygel®, EryDerm®, Staticin® Erymax®, Erythra-Derm® Generics available Pregnancy: B or C; Lactation: Unsafe **Gel, topical 2%:** 30 mL	**Adolescent and Adult gel and topical solution:** Apply twice daily after cleansing. May see response in 3-8 weeks; however, may require 12 weeks for full response. Continue as long as satisfactory response is maintained and side effects do not occur. **Important side effects:** May cause irritation, drying, pruritus, erythema. **Caution:** Avoid contact with eye(s) and mucous membranes.

Drug	Typical Dosing
Solution, topical 1.5% and 2% **Ointment, topical 2%:** 25 gm **Pledgets:** 2%	
Erythromycin Ophthalmic* Ilotycin® Generics available Pregnancy: B; Lactation: Safe **Ophthalmic ointment 0.5%**	**Children and Adult:** Apply 0.5-1 cm ribbon to lower conjunctival sac and gently massage eyelid. After 1 minute, excess ointment may be gently wiped away with sterile gauze. Repeat one or more times daily depending upon infection.
Famciclovir Famvir® Pregnancy: B; Lactation: Unsafe **Tabs:** 125 mg 250 mg 500 mg	**Children:** Safety and efficacy in children have not been established. **Adult:** 125 mg PO every 12 hours to 500 mg PO every 8 hours. **Food:** May be taken without regard to food. **Important side effects:** Nausea, diarrhea, headache, dizziness, insomnia, fatigue, rash. **Reduce dose in renal disease:** If usual dose is 500 mg PO every 8 hours and: CrCl 40-59 mL/min, then use 500 mg PO every 12 hours CrCl 20-39 mL/min, then use 500 mg PO every 24 hours CrCl <20 mL/min, then use 250 mg PO every 48 hours If usual dose is 125 mg every 12 hours and: CrCl 20-39 mL/min, then use 125 mg every 24 hours CrCl <20 mL/min, then use 125 mg every 48 hours
Fluconazole* Diflucan® Pregnancy: C; Lactation: Unsafe **Tabs:** 50 mg 100 mg	**Children ≥6 months to 13 years:** **Oropharyngeal candidiasis:** 6mg/kg/day on day 1 (max 200 mg), followed by 3 mg/kg/day (max 100 mg) thereafter. **Adult:** 100-400 mg PO onco daily. **Food:** May be taken without regard to food.

(continued)

Drug	Typical Dosing
150 mg 200 mg **Powder for Oral Suspension:** 10 mg/mL 40 mg/mL	**Important side effects:** Dizziness, headache, rash (may be severe), nausea, vomiting, diarrhea, abdominal pain, elevated LFTs. **Caution:** May cause elevated LFTs and hepatitis. Advise patient to contact provider if prodromal signs of liver dysfunction occur, i.e., abdominal pain, yellowing of skin or eye(s), unusual tiredness, dark urine, or pale stools. **Reduce dose in renal disease.** In patients with CrCl≤ 50 mL/min, give usual dose once, then 50% of dose at regular intervals thereafter. **Drug interactions may be significant, including:** Oral hypoglycemic agents, warfarin, cyclosporine, zidovudine, cisapride, rifabutin, phenytoin, rifampin, benzodiazepines, tacrolimus, hydrochlorothiazide, corticosteroids, buspirone, tricyclic antidepressants, alfentanil, vinca alkaloids.
Gatifloxacin* Tequin® Pregnancy: C; Lactation: Unsafe **Tabs:** 200 mg 400 mg	**≥18 years to Adult:** 200-400 mg PO once daily. **Food:** May take without regard to food. Do not take within 4 hours of sucralfate, antacids, aluminum, magnesium, calcium, zinc, iron, vitamins, or mineral supplements. **Important side effects:** Photosensitivity, dizziness, headache, insomnia, rash (may be severe), seizures, superinfection. **Drug interactions may be significant, especially:** Cyclosporine, warfarin, theophylline. **Reduce dose in renal disease:** CrCl <40 mL/min give 400 mg once, then 200 mg daily thereafter.
Griseofulvin (microsize) Grifulvin V®, Fulvicin U/F®, Grisactin® Pregnancy: C; Lactation: Unk **Tabs:** 250 mg 500 mg	**Children ≥2 years:** 10-20 mg/kg/day in one or two divided doses (max 500 mg/day). **125 mg/5 mL @ 10 mg/kg/day** 5 kg (11 lb) = 2 mL Q24H 7.5 kg (16 lb) = 3 mL Q24H 10 kg (22 lb) = 4 mL Q24H 12.5 kg (28 lb) = 5 mL (1tsp) Q24H

Drug	Typical Dosing
Caps: 250 mg **Oral Suspension:** 125 mg/5 mL	15 kg (33 lb) = 6 mL Q24H 20 kg (44 lb) = 8 mL Q24H 25 kg (55 lb) = 10 mL (2tsp) Q24H or 250 mg tab/cap Q24H **Adult**: 500 mg PO once or twice daily. **Food:** Take with a fatty meal to improve absorption. Avoid alcohol. **Important side effects:** Nausea, vomiting, diarrhea, photosensitivity, rash, urticaria, confusion, granulocytopenia, dysgeusia, disulfiram-like reaction, hepatotoxicity. **May reduce the efficacy of oral contraceptives.** **Caution:** Avoid excessive sun exposure. May cause hypersensitivity in some persons with penicillin allergy, use with caution. May cause birth defects, do not use in pregnancy. Males should wait at least 6 months after therapy before fathering a child. Use with caution in persons with history of liver disease or SLE. **Significant drug interactions:** Oral contraceptives, anticoagulants, cyclosporine.
Griseofulvin (ultramicrosize) Fulvicin P/G®, Gris-PEG® Generics available Pregnancy: C; Lactation: **Tabs:** 125 mg 165 mg 250 mg 330 mg Griseofulvin ultramicrosize demonstrated better oral absorption than griseofulvin microsize, permitting lower doses. There is no evidence that this effects therapeutic outcome.	**Children ≥2 years:** 5-10 mg/kg/day in one or two divided doses (max 330 mg). **Adult:** 330-750 mg/day in one or two divided doses. **Food:** Take with a fatty meal to improve absorption. Avoid alcohol. **Important side effects:** Nausea, vomiting, diarrhea, photosensitivity, rash, urticaria, confusion, granulocytopenia, dysgeusia, disulfiram-like reaction, hepatotoxicity. **May reduce the efficacy of oral contraceptives.** **Caution:** Avoid excessive sun exposure. My cause hypersensitivity in some persons with penicillin allergy, use with caution. May cause birth defects; do not use in pregnancy. Males should wait at least 6 months after therapy before fathering a child. Use with caution in persons with history of liver disease or SLE. **Significant drug interactions:** Oral contraceptives, anticoagulants, cyclosporine.

(continued)

Drug	Typical Dosing
Hydrocortisone/Polymyxin B Otic Otobiotic® Pregnancy: Unk; Lactation: Unk **Otic Solution 0.5% HC:** (15 mL) - $23.29	**Adult:** Instill 4 drops in affected ear(s) 3 or 4 times daily.
Imiquimod Cream 5% Aldara Cream® Pregnancy: B; Lactation: Unk **Cream 5%:** 250 mg single use packets in box of 12 packets.	**Adult:** Apply with finger to the warts at bedtime three times a week. Gently rub in until cream is no longer visible. Leave on 6-10 hours during sleeping hours, and then gently wash area with soap and water. Continue until all warts have cleared or up to 16 weeks. Wash hands before and after application. **Important side effects:** Itching and burning. Erythema is common. Pain, erosions, ulceration, headache. Fungal infection. May take a rest period if needed to allow discomfort to subside. **May weaken latex condoms and diaphragms. Concurrent use is not recommended.** **Caution:** Avoid sexual contact while cream is on skin.
Itraconazole* Sporanox® Pregnancy: C; Lactation: Unsafe **Caps:** 100 mg **Oral Solution:** 100 mg/10 mL	**Children:** 5 mg/kg/day (max 100 mg/day) once daily for 4-6 weeks. **Limited information on use in children. Avoid if possible.** **Using 100 mg/10 mL @ 5 mg/kg/day** 5 kg (11 lb) = 2.5 mL Q24H 10 kg (22 lb) = 5 mL (1 tsp) Q24H 15 kg (33 lb) = 7.5 mL Q24H 25 kg (55 lb) = 10 mL (2 tsp) Q24H or 100-mg cap **Adult:** 100-600 mg/day in one to three divided doses (usual maximum 200 mg/dose). **Food:** Avoid grapefruit products while taking. Take capsules with food, and take oral solution on an empty stomach.

Drug	Typical Dosing
	Important side effects: Headache, dizziness, rash, vomiting, diarrhea, hypertension, hypokalemia, cardiac arrhythmias, elevated LFTs, hepatitis. Advise patient to report any prodromal signs of liver failure (fatigue, weakness, nausea, vomiting, yellowing of eye(s) or skin). **Caution:** May cause hepatitis. Use with caution in persons with history of liver disease. Consider periodic liver function tests. May cause or contribute to congestive heart failure or cardiac dysrhythmias. Use with caution in persons with history of cardiac disease. Use for onychomycosis is contraindicated in patients with history of ventricular dysfunction or CHF. Use is contraindicated in any patient taking cisapride, dofetilide, quinidine, midazolam, triazolam, pimozide, lovastatin, or simvastatin. Not well absorbed with acid-suppressing drug. Has caused bone defects and changes in tooth appearance in rats; implications for humans are not established. **Drug interactions may be common and significant, including**: Cisapride (avoid), alfentanil, benzodiazepines, buspirone, calcium channel blockers, carbamazepine, corticosteroids, cyclosporine, digoxin, dofetilide, haloperidol, HMG-CoA reductase inhibitors, phenytoin, oral hypoglycemics, pimozide (avoid), protease inhibitors, rifamycin, quinidine, tacrolimus, tolterodine, vinca alkaloids, warfarin, acid-suppressing drugs and antacids. Women of child-bearing age should use an effective form of contraception during and for 1 month after therapy.
Ketoconazole* Nizoral® Generics available Pregnancy: C; Lactation: Unsafe	**Children ≥2 years:** 3.3-6.6 mg/kg once daily (max 400 mg/day). **200 mg @ 4-5 mg/kg daily** 25 lb (11 kg) = ¼ tab Q24H 50 lb (22 kg) = ½ tab (2.5 mL) Q24H

(continued)

Drug	Typical Dosing
Tabs: 200 mg **Cream 2%:** (15, 30, 60 g) **Shampoo 2%**	75 lb (33 kg) = ¾ tab (7.5 mL) Q24H 100 lb (45 kg) = 1 tab (5 mL) Q24H **Adult:** 200-400 mg PO once daily. **Shampoo:** Dampen affected area and apply shampoo. Rinse thoroughly after 1 minute. Repeat 2 times a week. **Cream:** Apply to affected area once or twice daily. **Food:** May take without regard to food. May take with food if GI upset occurs. Avoid taking within 2 hours of acid-suppressing drugs. **Important side effects:** Headache, dizziness, nausea, vomiting, hepatotoxicity, rash, urticaria, pruritus, reduced testosterone levels, gynecomastia. Advise patient to report any prodromal signs of liver failure (fatigue, weakness, nausea, vomiting, yellowing of eye(s) or skin). Shampoo may take curl out of permanently styled hair. **Caution:** Has been associated with fatal hepatotoxicity; monitor liver function closely. **Drug interactions may be significant, including:** Antacids, didanosine, tricyclic antidepressants, carbamazepine, proton pump inhibitors, H2 blocking agents, quinidine, benzodiazepines, buspirone, sulfonylureas, oral contraceptives, donepezil, tacrolimus, cyclosporine, isoniazid, warfarin, corticosteroids, rifampin, theophylline. **Efficacy of oral contraceptives may be reduced, and ketoconazole has caused birth defects in animals. Advise women of child-bearing potential to use effective alternative birth control.**
Levofloxacin* Levaquin® Pregnancy: C; Lactation: Unk **Tabs:** 250 mg 500 mg 750 mg	**≥18 years to Adult:** 250-500 mg PO once daily. **Food:** May take without regard to food. Do not take within 2 hours of sucralfate, antacids, aluminum, magnesium, calcium, zinc, iron, vitamins, or mineral supplements. **Important side effects:** Photosensitivity, dizziness, headache, insomnia, rash (may be severe), seizures, superinfection.

Drug	Typical Dosing
	Reduce dose in renal disease: CrCl 20-49 mL/min Give 500 mg PO followed by 250 mg PO Q24H CrCl 10-19 mL/min Give 500 mg PO followed by 250 mg PO Q48H **Drug interactions may be significant, especially:** Cyclosporine, warfarin, theophylline.
Lindane 1% G-well®, Kwell® Generics available Pregnancy: B; Lactation: Unk **Lotion 1%:** (30 mL, 60 mL) (30-60 mL should be sufficient quantity for child ≥6 years to Adult for one application). **Shampoo 1%:** (30 mL, 60 mL)	**Shampoo (pediculosis):** **Children and Adults:** Apply 15-30 mL to dry hair and work in well. Allow to remain on hair for 4 minutes, then apply water and lather and rinse thoroughly. Avoid contact with eye(s) and other mucous membranes. Comb hair with fine-toothed nit comb to remove nits. Repeat in 7 days only if lice or nits are still seen. **Lotion (scabies):** **Children and Adult:** Apply a thin layer and massage well into skin from chin line to toes (head to toe in infants). Wash off after 6 hours (infant), 6-8 hours (child), 8-12 hours (adult). Do not repeat sooner than 1 week and only if live mites are seen. **Important side effects:** Nausea, vomiting, headache, and seizure may be signs of excessive absorption. Contact health care provider immediately. **Caution:** Do not apply after bathing or apply to extensive areas of dermatitis or to acutely inflamed, raw, or weeping skin. Use with caution in persons with history of seizure disorder, especially infants or young children. Do not use in pregnant or lactating women. Avoid contact with eye(s), face, mucous membranes, and urethra. Cover hands of infants to avoid ingestion.
Metronidazole* Flagyl® Generics available Pregnancy: B; Lactation: Unsafe	**Children:** Amebic infection: 35-50 mg/kg/day in divided doses three times daily (max 2250 mg/day). Other infections: 15-30 mg/kg/day in divided doses 3 or 4 times daily (max 4 g/day).

(continued)

Drug	Typical Dosing
Tabs: 250 mg 500 mg **Caps:** 375 mg **Tabs, Extended Release (ER):** 750 mg	**Adult:** 7.5 mg/kg every 6 hours (max 4 g/day). Usual dose 250-500 mg PO every 6 hours. **Food:** Administer on empty stomach. May take with food if GI upset occurs. **Important side effects:** Nausea, vomiting, diarrhea, metallic taste in mouth, headache, psychotic reactions, darkening of urine, seizures, peripheral neuropathy, disulfiram-like reaction with ethanol. No alcohol. **No need to adjust dose in renal disease.** **Reduce dose in patients with liver disease.** **Drug interactions may be significant, especially:** Ethanol, warfarin, phenytoin, barbiturates, disulfiram, and lithium.
Metronidazole Gel* MetroGel-Vaginal® Pregnancy: B; Lactation: Unsafe **Gel, vaginal 0.75%:** 70-g tube with applicator	**Adult:** Insert one applicator intravaginally once or twice daily for 5 days. For once-daily application, administer at bedtime. Avoid contact with eye(s). Do not engage in vaginal intercourse while using this product. **Important side effects:** Candidal vaginitis, vaginal irritation, headache, dizziness, bad taste, disulfiram-like reaction with ethanol.
Metronidazole Topical* MetroGel®, MetroLotion®, Noritate® Pregnancy: B; Lactation: Unsafe **Lotion 0.75%** **Cream 1%** **Gel 0.75%**	**Adult:** Apply a thin film to the affected area twice daily after washing. Avoid contact with eye(s). May apply cosmetics over metronidazole. Therapeutic effect should be seen within 3 weeks. **Important side effects:** Generally well tolerated. May cause transient stinging or burning. Use with caution in patients taking oral anticoagulants; may require adjustment of anticoagulant dose.
Moxifloxacin* Avelox® Pregnancy: C; Lactation: Unk **Tabs:** 400 mg	**≥18 years to Adult:** 400 mg PO once daily. **Food:** May take without regard to food. Must take 4 hours before or 8 hours after sucralfate, antacids, aluminum, magnesium, calcium, zinc, iron, vitamins, or mineral supplements.

Drug	Typical Dosing
	Important side effects: Photosensitivity, dizziness, headache, insomnia, rash (may be severe), seizures, superinfection. **Do not need to educe dose in renal disease.** **Caution:** May prolong QT interval. Avoid use in patient with uncorrected hypokalemia or those taking Class 1A (e.g., procainamide, quinidine) or Class III antiarrhythmic agents. **Drug interactions may be significant especially:** Cyclosporine, warfarin, theophylline.
Mupirocin* Bactroban® Pregnancy: B; Lactation: Unk **Ointment 2%** **Cream 2%** **Ointment, nasal 2%**	**Children and adult:** Apply cream or ointment to affected area three times daily. **Nasal:** Apply half of each 1-g tube to each nostril two times daily for 5 days. After application, press together sides of nostrils and release, repeating for 1 minute to spread ointment. **Important side effects:** Burning, stinging, itching, headache. Nasal: rhinitis, upper respiratory congestion, pharyngitis, taste perversion.
Nitrofurantoin* Macrodantin®, Furadantin®, Macrobid® Generics available Pregnancy: B; Lactation: Safe **Caps:** 25 mg 50 mg 100 mg **Macrobid®:** 100 mg **Oral Suspension:** 25 mg/5 mL 60 mL	**Children ≥1 month:** 5-7 mg/kg/day in divided doses every 6 hours (max 400 mg/day). UTI prophylaxis 1-2 mg/kg/day as single dose (max 100 mg). **Adult:** 50-100 mg PO every 6 hours. **2.5/mg/kg/day** 10 kg (22 lb) = ¼ tsp Q6H 20 kg (44 lb) = ½ tsp (2.5 mL) Q6H 30 kg (66 lb) = 1 tsp (5 mL) Q6H **Food:** Take with food or milk. Maintain diet adequate in protein and vitamin B complex. **Important side effects:** May discolor urine. Nausea, vomiting, dizziness, headache, rash, hemolytic anemia, granulocytopenia, thrombocytopenia, hepatitis, jaundice, interstitial pneumonitis, fibrosis.

(continued)

Drug	Typical Dosing
	Caution: Contraindicated in women at term or in labor. Use with caution in G-6-PD deficiency, anemia, diabetes, or electrolyte abnormalities. Monitor for pulmonary or hepatic reactions or peripheral neuropathy. **Do not use in renal impairment. Ineffective if CrCl <40 mL/min.**
Nystatin* Mycostatin®, Nilstat® Generics available Pregnancy: B; Lactation: Unk **Oral Suspension:** 100,000 U/mL **Troche:** 200,000 U **Oral tablets:** 500,000 U This product is not for routine treatment of oral thrush.	**Newborns:** 100,000 U/mL – ½ mL in each cheek four times daily for 10-14 days. **Infants:** 100,000 U/mL – 1 mL in each cheek four times daily for 10-14 days. **Children:** 100,000 U/mL – 3 mL in each cheek four times daily **or** 1-2 pastilles four to five times a day for 10-14 days. **Adult:** 4-6 mL swish/swallow four times daily **OR** 1-2 pastilles four to five times a day for 10-14 days. **Retain in mouth as long as possible. Pastilles should be dissolved slowly.** **Important side effects:** Diarrhea.
Nystatin* Generics available Pregnancy: B; Lactation: Unk **Tablet, vaginal:** 100,000 U (15's and 30's with applicator) 15's - $32.30	**Adolescent and Adult:** Insert one tablet high in the vagina every night at bedtime for 2 weeks.
Nystatin* Mycostatin®, Nilstat® Generics available Pregnancy: B; Lactation: Safe **Cream 100,000 U/g** **Ointment 100,000 U/g**	**Children and Adult:** Apply to affected area two or three times daily after washing and drying. **Important side effects:** Well tolerated.

Drug	Typical Dosing
Ofloxacin* Floxin® Pregnancy: C; Lactation: Unk **Tabs:** 200 mg 300 mg 400 mg **Ophthalmic solution**	**≥18 years to Adult:** 200-400 mg PO every 12 hours. **Food:** May take without regard to food. Do not take within 2 hours of sucralfate, antacids, aluminum, magnesium, calcium, zinc, iron, vitamins, or mineral supplements. **Important side effects:** Photosensitivity, dizziness, headache, insomnia, rash (may be severe), seizures, superinfection. **Reduce dose in renal disease:** CrCl 20-50 mL/min give usual dose Q24H CrCl <20 mL/min give ½ usual dose Q24H **Drug interactions may be significant, especially:** Cyclosporine, warfarin, theophylline.
Penicillin V Potassium Pen-Vee K® Veetids® Generics available Pregnancy: B; Lactation: Unk **Tabs:** 250 mg 500 mg **Powder for Oral Suspension:** 125 mg/5 mL 250 mg/5 mL	**Children <12 years:** 25-50 mg/kg/day in divided doses every 6 to 8 hours (max 3 g/day) **125 mg/5 mL @ 25 mg/kg/day** 10 kg (22 lb) = ½ tsp (2.5 mL) Q6H 15 kg (33 lb) = ¾ tsp Q6H 20 kg (44 lb) = 1 tsp (5 mL) Q6H >20 kg (44 lb) = Use adult dose. **250 mg/5 mL @ 50 mg/kg/day** 10 kg (22 lb) = ½ tsp (2.5 mL) Q6H 15 kg (33 lb) = ¾ tsp Q6H 20 kg (44 lb) = 1 tsp (5 mL) Q6H >20 kg (44 lb) = Use adult dose. **Children ≥12 years to Adult:** 125-500 mg PO every 6 to 8 hours. **Food:** Take 1 hour before or 2 hours after meals. May take with food if GI upset occurs. **Important side effects:** Bad taste, GI upset, vomiting, diarrhea, agitation, seizures, rash, bleeding abnormalities, decreased WBC count, drug fever, superinfection.

(continued)

Drug	Typical Dosing
	Caution: Avoid use in patients with history of severe penicillin allergy. Use with caution in patients with history of seizures. **Do not need to adjust dose in renal disease.**
Permethrin Nix Cream Rinse® 1% Elimite® 5% Pregnancy: B; Lactation: Unk **Cream Rinse 1% (OTC)** **Cream 5%:** (**Note:** This product is for scabies, not for lice.)	**Cream Rinse 1%:** **Children ≥2 months to Adult:** Rinse: Wash hair, towel dry, saturate hair with Nix, rinse after 10 minutes. Remove remaining nits with nit comb. One treatment eliminates infestations. Repeat only if live lice are seen after 7 days. Wash bedding and all clothing. Vacuum furniture and dispose of bag. **Cream 5% (Scabies):** **Children ≥2 months to Adult:** Massage into all areas of skin from chin line to toe (head to toe in infants), leave on for 8-14 hours, then wash off thoroughly. May repeat in 1 week if live mites are seen. **Important side effects:** Mild temporary itching or erythema. **Caution:** Avoid contact with mucous membranes. Contraindicated if allergic to chrysanthemum flower.
Podofilox Condylox® Pregnancy: C; Lactation: Unsafe **Topical Solution 0.5%:** Indicated for external genital warts only, not for perianal or mucous membrane application. 3.5 g - $110.53 **Topical Gel 0.5%:** Indicated for external genital and perianal warts, not for mucous membrane application.	**Adults:** Apply minimal amount to cover wart with cotton tipped applicator Q12H for 3 days, then none × 4 days. Allow to air dry before contact with opposing skin or clothing. Wash hands before and after use. Repeat weekly until no warts are seen or up to 4 weeks. **Important side effects:** Burning, pain, itching, inflammation, erosion, bleeding. **Caution: Avoid contact with eye(s):** If eye(s) contact occurs, flush with water immediately and seek medical evaluation.

Drug	Typical Dosing
Polymyxin B + trimethoprim* Polytrim® Pregnancy: C; Lactation: Unk **Ophthalmic solution**	**Children ≥2 months to Adult:** Instill 1 drop in the effects eye(s) every 3 hours (max 6 drops/eye(s)/day). **Important side effects:** Redness, burning, stinging, itching.
Pyrethrins/piperonyl butoxide (OTC) RID®, A-200®, Pronto® Others available Pregnancy: C; Lactation: Unk 60-, 120-, 240-mL bottles 120 mL = 2 applications	**Children and Adult:** Apply to dry hair. After 10 minutes, wash hair, rinse thoroughly. Comb out hair with nit comb. Repeat 7-10 days. Wash bedding and all clothing. Vacuum furniture and dispose of bag. **Important side effects:** Burning, pruritus. **Caution:** Contraindicated if allergic to ragweed or chrysanthemum flower.
Selenium sulfide* Selsun®, Excel® Generics available Pregnancy: C; Lactation: Unk **Shampoo:** Selsun Blue® 1% (OTC) **Shampoo and Lotion:** 2.5% (120, 240 mL)	**Children and Adult:** Shampoo twice weekly until resolved (average 2 weeks). Leave in hair for 2-3 minutes, then rinse and repeat. Wash hands after use. Avoid contact with eye(s) and inflamed skin. **Important side effects:** May irritate skin and discolor hair or jewelry. Rinse thoroughly after use.
Spectinomycin Trobicin® Pregnancy: B; Lactation: Unknown **Powder for IM injection:** 2 g vial with 3.2 mL diluent (400 mg/mL when reconstituted)	**Children <45 kg:** 40 mg/kg IM once (max 2 g). **Children ≥45 kg to Adult:** 2 g IM once. Multiple doses may be required in disseminated gonococcal infection. **Important side effects:** Pain at injection site, dizziness, nausea, urticaria.

(continued)

Drug	Typical Dosing
Sulfacetamide sodium* Bleph-10®, Sulamyd® Sodium Sulamyd® Generics available Pregnancy: C; Lactation: Unsafe **Ophthalmic solution 10%, 15%, and 30%** **Ophthalmic Ointment 10%**	**Children ≥2 months to Adult:** **Ophthalmic solution 10%:** Instill 1-2 drops in the lower conjunctival sac of affected eye(s) every 1 to 3 hours while awake, less often at night. Frequency depends on severity of infection. **Ophthalmic ointment 10%:** Apply a ribbon to the lower conjunctival sac four times daily and at bedtime. May also use at bedtime in addition to solution during daytime. 30% solution should be used for severe infections only. **Important side effects:** Burning, sensitivity to light, headache, rash, hypersensitivity, bone marrow suppression, blurred vision. **Caution:** Use with caution in persons with G-6-PD deficiency or dry eye(s).
Terbinafine Lamisil® Pregnancy: B; Lactation: Unsafe **Tabs:** 250 mg **Cream 1%** **Topical Gel 1%**	**Children: Difficult to give to children <20 kg.** **<20 kg:** 62.5 mg once daily for 4 to 8 weeks. **20-40 kg:** 125 mg once daily for 4 to 8 weeks. **≥40 kg and Adult:** 250 mg PO Q24H **Food:** May take with or without meals. **Important side effects:** Ocular changes, rash, neutropenia, hepatobiliary dysfunction, nausea. Advise patient to report any prodromal signs of liver failure (fatigue, weakness, nausea, vomiting, yellowing of eye(s) or skin, dark urine, pale stools). **Caution:** Liver failure and death have occurred. Baseline LFTs should be obtained, and use of the drug should be avoided in persons with preexisting liver disease. **Avoid use in liver or renal (CrCl <50 mL/min) disease.** **Topical:** Apply to affected area once or twice daily until clinical signs and symptoms are significantly improved, a minimum 1 week, but no longer than 4 weeks. Avoid eye(s) and mucous membranes. Avoid occlusive dressings. **Important side effects:** Irritation, burning.

Drug	Typical Dosing
Tetracycline* Sumycin®, Tetracap® Generics available Pregnancy: D; Lactation: Unsafe **Caps:** 100 mg 250 mg 500 mg **Tabs:** 250 mg 500 mg **Oral Suspension:** 125 mg/5 mL	**Children ≥8 years:** 25-50 mg/kg/day in divided doses four times daily (max 3 g/day). **Adolescent and Adult:** 250-500 mg PO two to four times daily. **Food:** Take 1 hour before or 2 hours after meals. Take with full glass of water to minimize esophagitis. Do not take within 3 hours of antacids, iron, milk, or other dairy or calcium products. **Important side effects:** Photosensitivity (use sunscreen), esophagitis. May discolor fingernails. Rash, nausea, vomiting, diarrhea, superinfection, hepatitis, damage to developing bones and teeth, renal damage. **Outdated tetracyclines are toxic and should not be used.** **Reduce dose in liver disease or renal disease:** CrCl 50-80 mL/min administer usual dose every 8-12 hours. CrCl 10-50 mL/min administer usual dose every 12-24 hours. CrCl <10 mL/min administer usual dose every 24 hours.
Trimethoprim/Sulfamethoxazole Bactrim®, Septra®, Cotrim® Generics available Pregnancy: C; Lactation: Unsafe **Tabs:** **Single Strength (SS):** 80 mg/400 mg **Double Strength (DS):** 160 mg/800 mg **Oral Suspension:** 40 mg/200 mg/5 mL	**Children ≥2months:** 6-12 mg/kg/day (TMP component) in divided doses twice daily (max 320 mg/day). **40 mg/200 mg/5 mL @ 8 mg/kg/day** 10 kg (22 lb) = 1 tsp (5 mL) PO Q12H 20 kg (44 lb) = 2 tsp (10 mL) or 1 SS Tab PO Q12H 30 kg (66 lb) = 3 tsp or 1 tbsp (15 mL) or 1½ SS Tab PO Q12H 40 kg (88 lb) = 4 tsp (20 mL) or 2 SS Tabs or 1 DS PO Q12H **Adult:** 1 DS tab PO Q12H **Food:** May be taken without regard to food. **Maintain good hydration.** **Important side effects:** Photosensitivity, rashes, nausea, headache, diarrhea, dizziness, hypersensitivity reactions (possibly severe), renal dysfunction, hyperkalemia, bone marrow suppression.

(continued)

Drug	Typical Dosing
	Caution: Severe or fatal rashes, hepatic effects and hematologic effects have occurred. Encourage patient to report **any** side effects. Educate the patient regarding signs of granulocytopenia or thrombocytopenia. Do not use at term in pregnant patients. Use with caution in G-6-PD deficiency or liver disease. **Drug interactions may be significant, including:** Warfarin, cyclosporine, phenytoin, methotrexate, sulfonylureas, zidovudine, and digoxin. **Reduce dose in renal failure:** CrCl 15-30 mL/min give ½ usual dose. CrCl <15 mL/min avoid use.
Valacyclovir Valtrex® Pregnancy: B; Lactation: Unk **Tabs:** 500 mg 1,000 mg	**Children:** Safety and efficacy in children have not been established. **Adult:** 500 mg PO 2 times daily to 1 g three times daily. **Food:** May be taken without regard to food. **Maintain good hydration.** **Important side effects:** Nausea, headache, diarrhea, dizziness, renal dysfunction, HUS/TTP. **Reduce dose in renal disease:** If usual dose is 1 g every 8 hours and: CrCl 30-49 mL/min, then use 1 g every 12 hours CrCl 10-29 mL/min, then use 1 g every 24 hours CrCl <10 mL/min, then use 500 mg every 24 hours If usual dose is 500 mg every 12 hours and: CrCl <30 mL/min, then use 500 mg every 24 hours To monitor maternal–fetal outcomes in pregnancy, Glaxo Wellcome maintains a Valacyclovir in Pregnancy Registry which physicians are encouraged to call: (800)-722-9292 ext: 58465.

Drug	Typical Dosing
Vancomycin Oral (Vancocin®) Generic Available Pregnancy: C; Lactation: Unsafe **Pulvules:** 125 mg, 250 mg **Powder for oral solution:** 1 g (provides 250 mg/5 mL), 10 g (provides 500 mg/6 mL)	**Children:** 40 mg/kg/day (max 2000 mg/day) PO in divided doses every 6 hours. **Adolescent and Adult:** 500-2000 mg/day in divided doses PO every 6-8 hours. Usual dose is 125 mg PO every 6 hours. **Important side effects:** Oral vancomycin is generally well tolerated and not well absorbed systemically. However, significant absorption may occur in some patients, especially those with active colitis and significant renal dysfunction.

(continued)

Centers for Disease Control Recommended Childhood Immunization Schedule

	Age											
Vaccine	**Birth**	**1 mo**	**2 mos**	**4 mos**	**6 mos**	**12 mos**	**15 mos**	**18 mos**	**24 mos**	**4-6 y**	**11-12 y**	**13-18 y**
Hepatitis B	Hep B #1	Hep B #2			Hep B #3				Hep B Series Catch-up			
Diphtheria, Tetanus, Pertussis			DTaP	DTaP	DTaP		DTaP			DTaP	Td	
***Haemophilus influenzae* type b**			Hib	Hib	Hib	Hib						
Inactivated Polio			IPV	IPV	IPV					IPV		
Measles, Mumps, Rubella						MMR #1				MMR #2	MMR Catch-up	
Varicella						Varicella			Varicella Catch-up			
Pneumococcal			PCV	PCV	PCV	PCV						

More information and recommendations can be found at: http://www.cdc.gov/nip/

Index